Workbook to Accompany

INTRODUCTION TO

NURSING ASSISTING:

Building Language Skills

RITA FREY, RN, M.A.T.
Bunker Hill Community College, Boston, MA

LISA SHEARER COOPER, B.A., M.A.

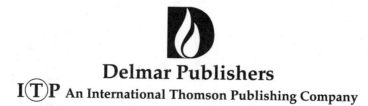

Delmar Publishers

I(T)P **An International Thomson Publishing Company**

Albany • Bonn • Boston • Cincinnati • Detroit • London • Madrid • Melbourne
Mexico City • New York • Pacific Grove • Paris • San Francisco • Singapore • Tokyo
Toronto • Washington

NOTICE TO THE READER

Cover Credit: Publisher Studio, Linda Ayres-DeMasi

COPYRIGHT © 1996
By Rita Frey and Lisa Shearer Cooper

The ITP logo is a trademark under license.

Printed in the United States of America

For more information, contact:

Delmar Publishers
3 Columbia Circle
Box 15015
Albany, New York 12212-5015

International Thomson Editores
Campos Eliseos 385, Piso 7
Col Polanco
11560 Mexico D F Mexico

International Thomson Publishing Europe
Berkshire House 168-173
High Holborn
London, WC1V7AA
England

International Thomson Publishing GmbH
Königswinterer Strasse 418
53227 Bonn
Germany

Thomas Nelson Australia
102 Dodds Street
South Melbourne, 3205
Victoria, Australia

International Thomson Publishing Asia
221 Henderson Road
#05-10 Henderson Building
Singapore 0315

Nelson Canada
1120 Birchmount Road
Scarborough, Ontario
Canada M1K5G4

International Thomson Publishing Japan
Hirakawacho Kyowa Building, 3F
2-2-1 Hirakawacho
Chiyoda-ku, Tokyo 102
Japan

1 2 3 4 5 6 7 8 9 10 XXX 02 01 00 99 98 97 96

Library of Congress Card Number: 95-45644

ISBN: 0-8273-6236-6

Delmar Publishers' Online Services

To access Delmar on the World Wide Web, point your browser to: http://www.delmar.com/delmar.html

To access through Gopher: gopher://gopher.delmar.com

(Delmar Online is part of "thomson.com", an Internet site with information on more than 30 publishers of the International Thomson Publishing Organization.)

For information on our products and services email: info@delmar.com or call 800-347-7707

Contents

Preface

This workbook has been written to complement the *Introduction to Nursing Assisting: Building Language Skills* textbook. The exercises and activities will help students master both the nursing assistant information and the English language.

Before beginning the exercises for each chapter, the student should read the Student Study Skills section, which includes information on using this book and the textbook. It also contains ideas on how to study, take notes, and make a schedule. The Student Study Skills section gives readers useful information to help them succeed as students.

Following the Student Study Skills section are short reviews of numbers and letters. Students taking this course should have studied this information before. However, if the information is not used, it is often forgotten. Correct use of numbers and letters is important for a nursing assistant student. These pages should be completed and mastered before moving on to the chapters.

The chapters are divided into topics that match the topics in the textbook. After completing one section of the textbook, the student may complete the matching section in the workbook. Some exercises may be done in class and others may be done as homework.

Student Study Skills

The key to being a good student is knowing how to study. Studying includes what you do daily in class and at home as well as preparing for examinations. In the following pages you will read ideas for making the most of your study time at school and at home. You will also learn ways to study for and take examinations.

STUDY SKILLS TO USE IN CLASS

Attendance

The first and most important thing to do is to be in class every day. Your instructor will have many ways to help you learn the information from the book. You may see videos or films, work with your classmates, or practice skills. You cannot make up for missed class time at home by studying the book. Nursing assisting is a hands-on course and you must be in class to learn the required skills.

Listening

When you are in class you must listen carefully. Think about what the instructor says. Also pay attention to the questions asked by fellow students. It is easy to let your mind wander to thinking about what the instructor is wearing or what you have to do after class. To prevent your mind from wandering you can start visualizing, or seeing in your mind, what is being explained. Repeat in your mind what the instructor is saying. You may also think of questions about anything that is not clear to you.

Asking Questions

Do not be afraid to ask questions. If you have a question, somebody else in the class probably has the same question. The instructor is there to answer your questions and help you understand. Help her do her job by asking questions when you do not understand something. Instructors are usually happy when students ask questions because it shows that the students are listening and trying to learn.

Taking Notes

Taking notes is an important skill for students. You may already have a method of note taking that works well for you. The most important thing is that the notes you take make sense to you when you read them later. You cannot, and do not want to, write down everything the instructor says. You need to pick out the main points and key words. If you have trouble knowing what the main points are, try reading the chapter before class. Then you will be familiar with the main points.

After class go through your notes and organize them in a way that makes sense to you. If your notes are not meaningful to you, they will not be of much use. The key to making your notes meaningful is making the information your own. Simple copying of information does not do much to make the information stick in your brain. As you look at the information, think it through and organize it.

Outlining. Outlining is one way to organize your notes. First, list the chapter title at the top. Then comes the first main point labeled with a Roman numeral I. Under that, list the information that goes with that title using a capital letter for each new point. Smaller bits of information are listed under the capital letters and are labeled with numbers, Figure 1.

STUDENT STUDY SKILLS

I. Study Skills to Use in Class

    A. Attendance

        1. Be there every day

        2. Many ways to learn information

            a. Films

            b. Work with classmates

            c. Practice Skills

        3. Cannot make up for missed class by studying at home

    B. Listening

        1. Focus on what is said.

        2. Do not let your mind wander.

        3. Ways to keep focused

            a. Visualize—see what is being said in your mind

            b. Repeat what the instructor says in your mind

            c. Form questions about parts that are unclear

    C. Asking Questions

        1. Do not be afraid ask

        2. Helps other students

        3. Helps instructor

Figure 1 This outline for the first part of the Student Study Skills shows how each smaller point is indented below a larger topic.

Mapping.　Another method of organizing your notes is with mapping. When mapping, you put the chapter title or main topic in a circle in the middle of the page. Then you draw lines out from it and write the smaller topics in smaller circles. From the smaller circles you draw a line for each bit of information that goes with the circle, Figure 2.

Colors.　Some people find it is helpful to use different colors for each topic. If you remember colors well you may want to try this method of making the information your own.

Working with Other Students

Get to know the other students in your class. Talking to them about the course is a good way to learn. Sometimes they may understand something you are having trouble with. Or you may be able to answer some of their questions. Either way you will be reinforcing, or making stronger, the new things you are learning. Having a study group to meet with before or after class is a great way to prepare for class or review new information. Knowing your classmates and feeling comfortable with them helps everybody learn more and enjoy the class.

Using Tape Recordings

If you have trouble understanding everything that is said in class you may wish to bring a small tape recorder to class with you. You may ask your instructor if you can record what is said in class and listen to it again later. Do this only if your instructor has said that it is all right to do so. Or, you may make your own recording of important information from the book and your notes. Having a recording gives you the chance to listen to it over and over. For some people this is a good way to learn. As with all of the methods for learning you need to try them to see what works for you.

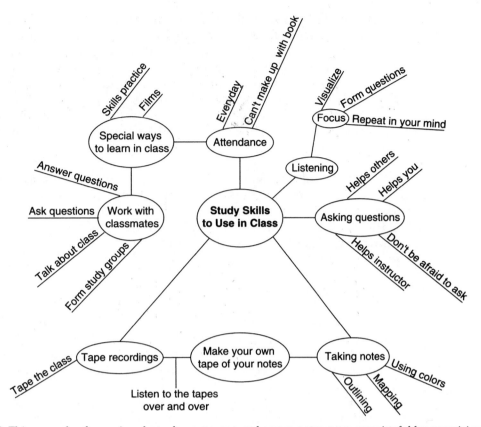

Figure 2 This example of mapping shows how you can make your notes more meaningful by organizing them. Notice how the item on "make your own tape of your notes" is linked to 2 topics.

STUDY SKILLS TO USE OUTSIDE OF CLASS

To study at home you need a work space and good light. If you have a desk that you use only for studying that is great. But a kitchen table works fine. You should have a regular place to keep your books and papers so you can find everything when you want to study. Routinely studying at the same time and place can help you remember things better. Some people study best with quiet. Others do better with music on. You will know what works best for you.

When studying with a tape you will need a quiet place so you can hear well. Or you may find you can concentrate better with earphones. Using earphones and a portable tape player will allow you to listen to the tapes while you do other things like riding the bus or walking.

Using the Book

The book is written to make learning easier for you. If the book belongs to you, you should feel free to write in the margins or to highlight sections that are important. Special markers allow you to color parts of the page and still be able to read the writing. Making the book your own by adding your comments and questions will help you learn the information.

The book has many features to help you study. At the end of each section are Stop and Think questions. Take time to answer these questions either in your mind or in your notebook. Some of the questions can be answered by looking back at the section. Other questions will require you to think about what you have read and then use it in some way. The "thinking" questions are more difficult but will teach you to use the information you are learning in the ways you will have to use it as a nursing assistant.

End of Chapter Study Tools. At the end of each chapter you will find many study tools. The first is the Language at Work dialogue. Here you will find a conversation based on the chapter you have just finished. A taped version of the conversation allows you to hear the sounds of the spoken language.

The Chapter Review allows you to check your understanding of the entire chapter. You may wish to study the chapter first and then see if you can answer the questions without looking back at the book. Or you can find the answers you do not know in the book as you go along. These exercises are like a self-test. The answers are provided so you can check your own work.

End of the Book Study Tools. At the end of the book are appendices that are included for your information and review. It is a good idea to look at these before beginning your studies so you know what is there. Also at the end is the glossary, which lists all the vocabulary words in the book and their meanings. Use it to check the meaning of a word quickly and easily. The index of the book gives the page number of topics and words in the book.

Using the Workbook and Tapes

The Workbook. The workbook is designed to give you further practice in the skills needed to be a nursing assistant. At the beginning of each chapter in the workbook you will find a list of the vocabulary and abbreviations for the chapter. Use these to check your knowledge. Try to define each item, then check your answers in the glossary at the back of the textbook.

Some of the exercises can be done at home. Others will be done in class. All of the activities will help strengthen what you have learned from the book and in class.

The Audio Tapes. The tapes may be used at home or at school. They have the pronunciation of vocabulary words for you to listen to and practice. They also have readings of the vocabulary sentences that are listed in the workbook. These readings allow you to hear vocabulary words used in the language instead of alone.

The pronunciation and listening exercises from the workbook are recorded on the tape so you can do the exercises in class or on your own. The Language at Work conversations are also recorded on the tapes. Pay attention to the melody or intonation of the sentences as well as the rhythm. Practice imitating these sounds.

How Can I Find Time to Study?

Studying for a long time every night is not necessary to learn new information. Once you have your notes organized, a simple reading of them before bed and again in the morning is often better than hours of trying to force the information into your brain. Spending 10 minutes before bed and 10 minutes in the morning every day may be more helpful than staying up all night once a week.

Time Management. You do need to find time to read the book, do the exercises, and organize your notes. If you are working, are a parent, or both, it can be hard to find enough hours in the day. Time management can help you schedule your day so you have time for the most important things. Fill out the schedule in Figure 3 with your weekly schedule.

Look for spaces of unused time that you can schedule as time for studying. Some students find they study well on the bus or train. Others use the breaks they are given at school. By following your schedule you will have a regular time for studying.

	Sunday	Monday	Tuesday	Wednesday	Thursday	Friday	Saturday
6:00 AM							
7:00							
8:00							
9:00							
10:00							
11:00							
12:00							
1:00 PM							
2:00							
3:00							
4:00							
5:00							
6:00							
7:00							
8:00							
9:00							
10:00							

Figure 3 Use this form to schedule your week so you have time for all the most important things in you life, including studying.

Studying When You Have Children. Parents often have trouble finding time to study at home. Here are some ideas to help you find time.

- If you have school-age children you may be able to set up a time when you all do your homework. Your studying may get interrupted when your children need help, but mostly it will be a quiet time for everyone to get school work done.
- Younger children may be kept busy with crayons and paper or a notebook of their own so they can "study" like you do.
- You may wish to use the time your children spend watching educational television programs as your study time.
- If you need absolute quiet to study you may need to ask another family member to take the children out for a while. You may need to explain to all family members the importance of your studying so they will cooperate in helping you find study time.
- You may wish to study at the school library before you go home if you find you cannot concentrate at home.
- Studying when children are asleep is a good way to have uninterrupted quiet time. You can study after they have gone to bed or before they get up in the morning.

STUDYING FOR AND TAKING TESTS

Studying for Tests

If you have followed good study habits from the beginning, much of your test preparation will already be done. You will study from your notes and book. Read through your notes and the highlights of your book. The best time to study is right before bed. Read the most important things to remember right before you sleep and again when you get up in the morning.

Memory Aids. If there are sets of information you need to memorize you can help yourself by using memory aids. One memory aid is to count the number of items in a set. Then when you try to remember them you will know if you've forgotten one. For example, in this course you will be learning many skills. Each skill has a number of steps to remember. When you know that a skill has 5 steps, you can count off how many steps you remember. If you remember only 3, you know you have 2 more to think of.

Another memory aid is called visualization. If you remember things by "seeing" them in your mind this may be a good memory aid for you. When you have something to remember, you make a picture of it in your mind. If you are trying to remember the steps of a procedure, you would "see," or visualize, yourself doing each step in your mind. Check your visualization with the book to make sure you visualized everything correctly. Then when it is time for the test you can close your eyes and visualize the procedure.

Visualization can also help you with spelling if that is a difficult area for you. You can visualize the word in your mind, carefully "writing" each letter. Notice the shape of the word, where it goes up and down, and how long it is. Always check your visualization with the book to make sure it is correct or you will remember it incorrectly.

Test Taking

Test taking is a skill that you will get better at as you take more and more tests. But there are things you can do to improve your test taking skills. The first is to study for the test ahead of time. No test-taking skills will save you if you do not study the material. Immediately before taking the test you may want to quickly read through your notes or parts of your notes that you have trouble with. Breathe deeply and try to relax.

When you get your test look through the entire test to see how long it is and what kinds of questions there are. Do the parts that are easiest for you first. If you come to a question you do not know, skip it and come back to it later. If you are taking a multiple choice test, answer all of the questions, even if you are not sure of the answers. On most tests it is better to guess than to leave it blank. When you have completed the test, read through it to check for any accidental errors. Do not change answers unless you are absolutely sure that you made a mistake.

Test Anxiety. Test taking can make some people nervous and anxious. When we feel upset it is harder to think and sometimes our minds go blank. This is called "test anxiety," which can make students who know the information still fail a test. How can you prevent test anxiety? First of all, study ahead of time. On the day of the test do not spend all day thinking about the test. Try to have a normal day. When you arrive at class, do not talk to students who are worried and anxious about the test. Sit quietly and read through your notes one last time. The advice on test taking is good for everyone to follow.

Some people have trouble taking a written test but can answer questions if they are spoken. If this is true for you then you should talk to your instructor. It may be possible to have someone read the test to you and let you answer orally. There are different ways to show that you know the information.

THE ENGLISH ALPHABET

At some point you probably learned the alphabet as part of an English course. However, most people tend to forget the pronunciation of letters unless they use them often. As a nursing assistant you will be using the names of letters in abbreviations and in spelling names. Below you will find a list of letters and their pronunciation based on common English words. Next to each letter is a space where you may write the pronunciation of each letter in your own language to help you remember how to say it.

A _____	**ay** as in day	N _____	**en** as in enter
B _____	**bee**	O _____	**oh**
C _____	**see**	P _____	**pee** as in peek
D _____	**dee** as in deep	Q _____	**cue** as in cute
E _____	**ee** as in eel	R _____	**are**
F _____	**ef** as in left	S _____	**es** as in estate
G _____	**jee** as in jeep	T _____	**tea**
H _____	**ay-ch**	U _____	**you**
I _____	**I** or **eye**	V _____	**vee** as in veal
J _____	**jay**	W _____	**double you**
K _____	**kay**	X _____	**eks** as in extreme
L _____	**el** as in elbow	Y _____	**why**
M _____	**em** as in empty	Z _____	**zee** as in zebra

(*Note:* Americans do not say "zed" for the letter Z as some other English speakers do.)

NUMBER WORDS

Numbers		Handwritten	
1	one	*1*	*1*
2	two	*2*	*2*
3	three	*3*	*3*
4	four	*4*	*4*
5	five	*5*	
6	six	*6*	
7	seven	*7*	*7*
8	eight	*8*	
9	nine	*9*	
10	ten	*10*	
11	eleven		
12	twelve		
13	**thirteen**		
14	fourteen		
15	**fifteen**		
16	sixteen		
17	seventeen		
18	**eighteen**		
19	nineteen		
20	**twenty**		
30	**thirty**		
40	forty		
50	**fifty**		
60	sixty		
70	seventy		
80	eighty		
90	ninety		
100	one hundred		

(Boldface indicates irregular form.)

The following handwritten numbers will be misunderstood by Americans.

1 will be read as a seven.

1 will not be understood at all.

9 will be read as the letter g.

Chapter 1: Health Care in the United States

VOCABULARY

activities of daily living
acute illness
addicted
anesthesia
Cardiac Care Unit
chronic illness
client
clinic
disability
Emergency Department
extended
geriatric
hospital
immunization
inpatient
injured

institution or facility
Intensive Care Unit
Labor and Delivery
Laboratory
long-term
Maternity
Medical-Surgical
mental
Nursery
Obstetrics and
    Gynecology
Operating Room
Orthopedics
outpatient
patient
Pediatrics

physical fitness
Physical Therapy
population
Postanesthesia Care
    Unit
psychiatric
Radiology
Recovery Room
rehabilitation
resident
restorative
skilled
stable
surgery
X-ray

ABBREVIATIONS

ATU	addictions treatment unit	**OB-GYN**	obstetrics and gynecology
CCU	cardiac care unit	**OR**	operating room
ED	emergency department	**ortho**	orthopedics
ICU	intensive care unit	**PACU**	postanesthesia care unit
lab	laboratory	**pedi/peds**	pediatrics
L&D	labor and delivery	**pt**	patient
LTC	long-term care	**PT**	physical therapy
mat	maternity	**SNF**	skilled nursing facility
med-surg	medical-surgical	**rehab**	rehabilitation
NF	nursing facility	**RR**	recovery room
NSY	nursery	**X-ray**	radiology

HEALTH CARE INSTITUTIONS

Vocabulary Sentences

1. Nursing assistants often work at a health care **institution or facility.**
2. A baby or a child may receive an **immunization** at a regular checkup.
3. A patient with an **acute illness** is often cared for at a doctor's office or clinic.
4. A patient with a **chronic illness** may be able to live at home.

Listening

Circle the word you hear.

1. patience	patent	patient
2. resident	residence	residue
3. immunize	immunization	immunity
4. clinical	clinic	chronic
5. accurate	acute	actual
6. institutionalize	institute	institution

Discussion

1. Explain the difference between chronic and acute illnesses. What kinds of health care facilities care for people with chronic problems? with acute problems?

2. Exercising your body is a good way to avoid illness. What are some ways to improve your physical fitness?

HOSPITALS AND LONG-TERM CARE

Vocabulary Sentences

1. The operation was done while the patient was an **inpatient.**
2. The clinic sees many **outpatients** during the day.
3. **Rehabilitation** hospitals are a great help for people who have suffered serious injuries.
4. **Geriatric** patients are the main population cared for in long-term care facilities.
5. Sometimes people with physical or mental **disabilities** need regular medical care.
6. Nursing assistants often help residents with **activities of daily living.**
7. Every long-term care facility and home care agency must be concerned with the **restorative** care of its residents.

Matching

Match the description of the general hospital department to the abbreviation of the name of the department.

___1. CCU
___2. ER or ED
___3. ICU
___4. L&D
___5. lab

___ 6. mat
___ 7. med-surg
___ 8. Nursery
___ 9. OB-GYN
___10. OR

___11. ortho
___12. PT
___13. pedi or peds
___14. RR or PACU
___15. X-ray

a. floor with inpatients who have medical problems, such as stomach problems, or who have had surgery
b. floor where children are cared for
c. special unit where very sick patients who need a lot of nursing care stay
d. special unit where patients who have heart problems stay
e. department that takes care of patients who have had accidents or an illness that needs immediate treatment
f. department where mothers give birth to their babies
g. floor where new mothers stay for 1 or 2 days after giving birth
h. floor where the babies stay after they are born
i. floor where patients with problems with their bones and muscles stay
j. department where they take pictures of bones
k. department where tests are done on blood and other body fluids
l. department where an operation (surgery) is done
m. unit where the patient wakes up from anesthesia after surgery
n. department where the patient learns how to use his body again and becomes strong after having an accident or surgery
o. department that takes care of women who are going to have babies and of women's health problems

Activity

Name as many health care facilities in your community as you can. Look in the telephone book for more health care facilities in your area. When you have a list of 10 facilities classify them by type.

For each facility ask yourself the following questions:

- Is it an acute or chronic care facility?
- Is the facility for one special type of patient or health care problem?

When you finish your list compare it with your classmates' lists. See how many different kinds of health care facilities are present in your community.

LANGUAGE AT WORK

Kathy: Mary, what floor are you working on today?

Mary: The supervisor was going to put me on med-surg, but they needed me on maternity, so I went there.

Kathy: It must be nice to work with the new mothers and babies. Today I was working on the ortho floor. We were very busy.

Mary: Really? What was going on?

Kathy: Well, there were several patients who just came back from PACU. Other patients were going to the OR. Someone else had to be sent to X-ray. Another man was being sent to a rehab hospital.

Mary: I guess you did have a busy morning, Kathy. I have to take this blood sample to the lab now, so I'll see you at lunch.

Questions:

1. What floor is Mary working on today?

   _____

2. What kind of patients are on that floor?

   _____

3. What floor is Kathy working on today?

   _____

4. What kind of patients are on that floor?

   _____

5. What other departments does Kathy talk about?

   _____

6. Why is a patient sent to the rehab hospital?

   _____

7. What does the lab do?

   _____

Chapter 2: Working in a Health Care Institution

VOCABULARY

antibiotic
care plan
certified
chain of command
dentist
diagnosis
dose
geriatric

illegal
in-service
interdisciplinary team
odor
order
personal hygiene
physician
podiatrist

prescription
rotate
shift
shift differential
sick day
skills test
supervisor

ABBREVIATIONS

AM	morning	PA	physician's assistant
CNA	certified nursing assistant	PCA	patient care assistant
Dr.	doctor	PM	after noon
HHA	home health aide	PT	physical therapist
LPN	licensed practical nurse	RD	registered dietitian
LVN	licensed vocational nurse	RN	registered nurse
MD	medical doctor	RT	respiratory therapist
NA	nursing assistant	SW	social worker
NP	nurse practitioner		
OBRA	Omnibus Budget Reconciliation Act		

THE NURSING ASSISTANT AS PART OF THE HEALTH CARE TEAM

Vocabulary Sentences

1. The **interdisciplinary team** works together to improve the life and the health of the patient.
2. A **certified** nursing assistant has more job opportunities than a nursing assistant without a certificate.
3. The **diagnosis** for Ms. Chan is breast cancer.
4. When the doctor said I had strep throat, she gave me a **prescription** for an **antibiotic.**
5. I take 1 **dose** 4 times each day.
6. A **podiatrist** is not a general medical doctor.

The Health Care Team Crossword Puzzle

Write either the abbreviation or the full word in the spaces, Figure 2–1.

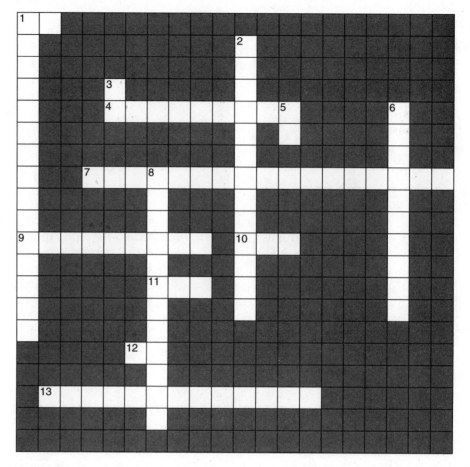

Figure 2–1

Across
1. Abbreviation for registered nurse
4. Makes out the food plan for the patient based on doctor's orders
7. Helps patient get stronger by having him do special exercises
9. Another name for nursing assistant
10. Abbreviation for certified nursing assistant
11. Abbreviation for licensed practical nurse
12. Abbreviation for doctor
13. Person who handles the telephone, written, and computer work on the floor

Down
1. A nurse with more education and responsibility than an LPN
2. Diagnoses and prescribes treatment for illnesses and has a 4-year medical degree
3. Abbreviation used after a name to show the person is a medical doctor
5. Abbreviation for nursing assistant
6. A doctor who takes care of feet
8. Helps patient with family or other nonmedical problems

ORGANIZATION OF NURSING CARE

Vocabulary Sentences

1. The **chain of command** lets everyone know to whom they report.
2. Mr. Zimmermann's **care plan** states that he needs to be fed at mealtime.
3. Part of the care plan is based on **orders** written by the doctor.
4. In some facilities nursing assistants work different **shifts** each month.
5. The **supervisor** gave instructions to the nurses and nursing assistants.

Role Play

Read the situation below. Then choose people to be Rebecca, Mohammed, and the nurse. Play the roles, acting out what they might say and how they might solve their problem. Part of the dialogue is written for you. Write in the other lines so that the conversations make sense.

Rebecca and Mohammed are nursing assistants at the medical center. Rebecca is new at the medical center and Mohammed has worked there for a year.

Mohammed is having a problem. When he is working, Rebecca tells him he is doing everything wrong. She says that she has learned to do it differently. Mohammed gets angry and walks away because he does not want to start an argument.

Rebecca is having a problem with Mohammed because she thinks that he is not careful enough in his work. When she tries to show him how to do the job correctly, he walks away. She feels that she has to do his work as well as her own work.

Rebecca: Mohammed, that is not the right way to make a closed bed. I will show you how to do it.

Mohammed:

Nurse: Mohammed, why are you walking down the hall with that angry look on your face? Has something happened?

Mohammed:

Nurse: Let me talk to Rebecca, and then later we will all talk together. Right now why don't you go see if Mr. Chavez needs anything.

_____

Nurse: Rebecca, I need to talk to you about Mohammed. Can you tell me what has been going on between the 2 of you?

Rebecca:

Nurse: Why don't you come with me, and we'll talk with Mohammed?

_____

Nurse: You 2 have been having some trouble. We work as a team at this hospital, so let's try to settle this problem. Rebecca, why don't you tell Mohammed how you felt about the situation.

Rebecca:

Nurse: Mohammed, tell Rebecca how you see the situation.

Mohammed:

Nurse: Is there some way we can work together on this?

Mohammed:

Rebecca:

Nurse: That sounds like a good way to solve the problem. And remember, if you are having a problem with each other, it's always best to talk to each other first. If you cannot solve the problem, then come talk to me.

Short Answer

Change the following times from the 12-hour clock to the 24-hour clock.

1. 6:00 AM   _____

2. 6:00 PM   _____

3. 11:35 AM   _____

4. 8:15 PM   _____

5. 12:40 AM   _____

6. 1:20 PM   _____

Change the following times from the 24-hour clock to the 12-hour clock.

1. 1627   _____

2. 2130   _____

3. 0830   _____

4. 0030   _____

5. 1230   _____

Write each of the times for the 3 normal shifts by the 12-hour clock and by the 24-hour clock.

Day: _____to_____   or _____to_____

Evening: _____to_____   or _____to_____

Night: _____to_____   or _____to_____

HOW TO PREPARE FOR YOUR JOB IN THE HEALTH CARE INSTITUTION

Writing

Write a paragraph in your own words about the importance of good personal hygiene and neat appearance of health care workers.

_____

_____

_____

_____

_____

_____

Matching

Match the hygiene behavior with how often you should do it. Some answers may be used more than once. Some answers may not be used at all.

For good hygiene you should:

___1. take a bath or shower
___2. brush your teeth
___3. wash your hair
___4. use deodorant or antiperspirant
___5. wear a fresh clean uniform
___6. go to the dentist

a. at least once a day
b. at least once a week
c. at least twice a day
d. at least twice a week
e. at least twice a year

LANGUAGE AT WORK

Kathy and Ali meet at the medical center. They were in a nursing assistant training course together.

Kathy: Hi, Ali. Are you working here at the medical center as a nursing assistant now?

Ali: Hello, Kathy. Yes, I've been working here for about a month.

Kathy: How do you like working at this center?

Ali: It's great. I'm so glad that I became a certified nursing assistant. The nurses and doctors are very nice here. There are a lot of new things to learn.

Kathy: What shift do you work?

Ali: I usually work the day shift, but sometimes I have to rotate to nights.

Kathy: Have you ever worked the evening shift?

Ali: Yes, for about 6 months when I was at a long-term care facility.

Kathy: What are your plans for the future?

Ali: I'd like to go to the community college and study to be a registered nurse.

Questions

1. At what kind of facility does Ali work?

   _____

2. How long has he been working there?

   _____

3. What shift does he work?

   _____

4. What would he like to do in the future? What kind of job would he like to have?

   _____

Chapter 3: Ethics in a Health Care Institution

VOCABULARY

abortion
abuse
advance directive
afford
assignment
cafeteria
call a code
capable
clergy
co-worker
confidential
damages

debt
dependable
discharged
donation
ethics
fired
gossip
handle
harm
health care proxy
legal

life-style
malpractice
negligence
organ transplants
personality
report
sue
technology
tip
trust
unconscious

ABBREVIATIONS

AMA against medical advice
DNR do not resuscitate
DRG diagnostic-related group

ETHICS FOR THE NURSING ASSISTANT

Vocabulary Sentences

1. **Ethics** are important in all parts of a person's life.
2. Every health care institution has its own way to **call a code.**
3. The hospital carries insurance to cover any **negligence** by its nursing assistants.
4. When you work on a floor you should help your **co-workers** whenever possible.
5. A nursing assistant must report **abuse** of an elderly person to the nurse.
6. All patient information is **confidential**.
7. Health care workers must be careful not to **gossip**.
8. The nurse told me to **report** to her when I finished my **assignment**.

Yes or No

Should a Nursing Assistant Do This? Read the following list to see which items a nursing assistant should do and which she should not do. If she should do it answer YES. If she should not do it answer NO.

_____1. Accept tips.

_____2. Be trustworthy.

_____3. Give medication.

_____4. Call a code when a patient stops breathing or his heart stops beating.

_____5. Discuss patient problems with the nurse on the floor.

_____6. Do a procedure she is not sure of.

_____7. Discuss patient problems with a nursing assistant friend from a different floor

_____8. Ask for help if unsure.

_____9. Tell a patient about your religion and try to make him believe the same as you do.

Writing

Look at the sentences above that you answered "NO." Choose one and write a paragraph about why a nursing assistant should not do it.

_____

_____

_____

_____

Role Play

The nurse asks the nursing assistant to do something for a patient that the nursing assistant has not done before. Choose 1 person to be the nurse and 2 students to be the nursing assistants. Continue the conversation started below.

Nurse: Pat, would you take Mr. McConnell to radiology please?

Pat:

Nurse: Oh, I didn't realize that you haven't been down there yet. Ask Marco to show you the way.

Pat:

Pat asks Marco if he has time to show her where the radiology department is.

Pat:

Marco:

(You may continue the conversation if you wish.)

PATIENTS' RIGHTS

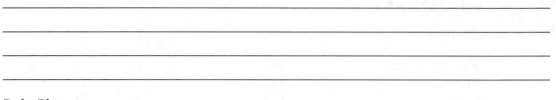

Vocabulary Sentences

1. An **advance directive** is sometimes called a living will.
2. Everyone is encouraged to sign a **health care proxy**.

Yes or No

Patients and residents have many rights that must be protected. Read each of the rights below. If it is a patient or resident right, write "YES" on the line. If it is not a patient right, write "NO" on the line.

_____1. To be free from restraints unless the restraint is absolutely necessary and ordered by the doctor

_____2. To be involved in making decisions about his care

_____3. To be free from abuse

_____4. To be told about the care he will receive

_____5. To make choices about his living conditions

_____6. To use his own clothing and other belongings

_____7. To have his privacy protected

_____8. To know how much the care costs

CURRENT ETHICAL QUESTIONS IN HEALTH CARE

Vocabulary Sentences

1. Patients often need home health care after they are **discharged** from the hospital.
2. **Organ transplants** can be done for people with heart, lung, or liver diseases.
3. **Abortion** is legal in the United States, but some people think it should be illegal.

Culture Exchange

Answer the questions below by yourself or with classmates from your country. Then find a partner from a different country and compare your answers.

1. How do people in your birth country pay for health care?

_____

_____

_____

_____

_____

2. Do people in your birth country have the same access to health care as people in the United States?

_____

_____

_____

_____

_____

3. Do people in your birth country have some medical treatments that people in the United States do not have?

_____

_____

_____

_____

_____

4. What are your thoughts and feelings about the differences in health care between your old country and your new country?

_____

_____

_____

_____

_____

Pronunciation

The letter "a" is pronounced in several different ways. Listen carefully as each word is pronounced. Repeat the word. Then place the word in the correct column.

damages
handle
AMA
malpractice
cafeteria
personality
capable

"a" in apple   "a" in f<u>a</u>ce

_____   _____

_____   _____

_____   _____

_____   _____

_____   _____

Discussion Questions

1. Explain the difference between an advance directive and a health care proxy. Tell how each affects medical care.

2. Are medical ethics in the United States the same as those in your country? How are they different? How do you feel about the differences?

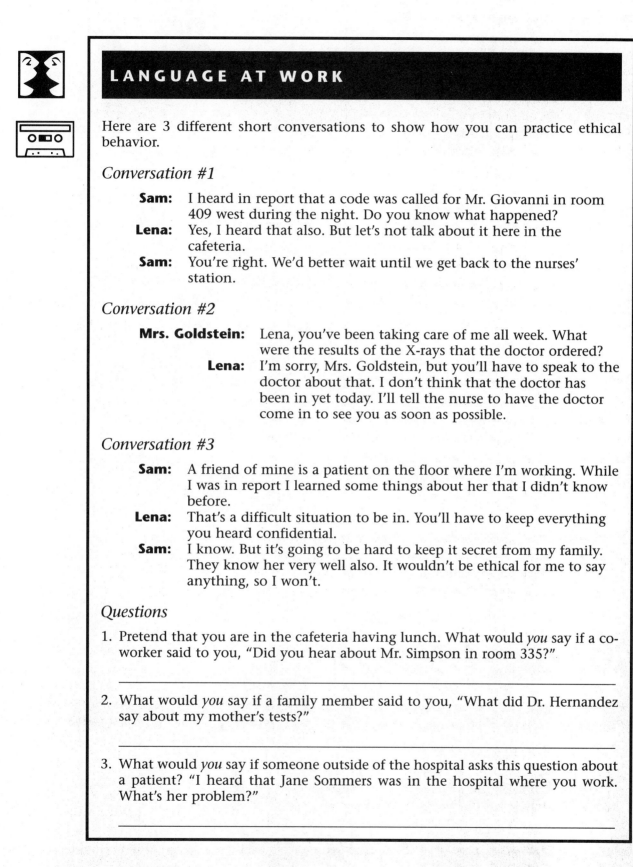

LANGUAGE AT WORK

Here are 3 different short conversations to show how you can practice ethical behavior.

Conversation #1

Sam: I heard in report that a code was called for Mr. Giovanni in room 409 west during the night. Do you know what happened?

Lena: Yes, I heard that also. But let's not talk about it here in the cafeteria.

Sam: You're right. We'd better wait until we get back to the nurses' station.

Conversation #2

Mrs. Goldstein: Lena, you've been taking care of me all week. What were the results of the X-rays that the doctor ordered?

Lena: I'm sorry, Mrs. Goldstein, but you'll have to speak to the doctor about that. I don't think that the doctor has been in yet today. I'll tell the nurse to have the doctor come in to see you as soon as possible.

Conversation #3

Sam: A friend of mine is a patient on the floor where I'm working. While I was in report I learned some things about her that I didn't know before.

Lena: That's a difficult situation to be in. You'll have to keep everything you heard confidential.

Sam: I know. But it's going to be hard to keep it secret from my family. They know her very well also. It wouldn't be ethical for me to say anything, so I won't.

Questions

1. Pretend that you are in the cafeteria having lunch. What would *you* say if a co-worker said to you, "Did you hear about Mr. Simpson in room 335?"

   _____

2. What would *you* say if a family member said to you, "What did Dr. Hernandez say about my mother's tests?"

   _____

3. What would *you* say if someone outside of the hospital asks this question about a patient? "I heard that Jane Sommers was in the hospital where you work. What's her problem?"

   _____

Chapter 4: Safety in a Health Care Institution

VOCABULARY

acquired immune
   deficiency
   syndrome
badge
blood-borne disease
body mechanics
call bell
choking
disaster
dispose of

document
emergency
environment
environmental services
hazard
identification bracelet
incident
intercom
life-threatening
nursing station

personal protection
   equipment
policy
prioritize
security personnel
sharps
splash
staff
violent
witness

ABBREVIATIONS

AIDS acquired immunodeficiency
       syndrome
HIV   human immunodeficiency virus
HBV hepatitis B virus
HCV hepatitis C virus

ID band identification bracelet
OSHA Occupational Safety and
        Health Administration
RACE Remove-Activate-Contain-
        Extinguish or Evacuate

KEEPING THE PATIENT SAFE

Vocabulary Sentences

1. When a patient enters a hospital she is given an **identification bracelet**.
2. Each patient has a **call bell** beside his bed.
3. Some call bells contain an **intercom** so that a patient can speak with someone at the **nursing station** immediately.
4. Pain around the heart is an example of a **life-threatening** problem.
5. Nursing assistants must learn to **prioritize** their duties.
6. If a patient falls out of bed, the nursing assistant must fill out an **incident** report.
7. It is important to **document** what happens to a patient.

Writing

Use your own words to make sentences using each of the following words.

1. intercom

_____

2. ID band

_____

3. life-threatening

_____

4. prioritize

_____

5. document

_____

6. witness

_____

7. emergency

_____

8. choking

_____

9. incident

_____

10. witness

_____

KEEPING THE NURSING ASSISTANT SAFE

Vocabulary Sentences

1. Protect yourself from back injuries by using good **body mechanics**.
2. **HIV** causes a **blood-borne disease** called **AIDS**.
3. **Personal protection equipment** helps protect health care workers from blood-borne diseases.
4. All **sharps** must be placed in special sharps containers immediately after they are used.
5. Nursing assistants must protect themselves from a **splash** that could spread hepatitis.

Role Play

Choose 2 nursing assistants, 2 patients, and 2 nurses to act out the following scenes. Act out what is written below and then continue the situation.

1. A nursing assistant in a long-term care facility goes to assist one of her regular residents with the morning activities of dressing and washing before breakfast. She knows this resident well and enjoys their morning conversations. When she knocks on the door and calls to the resident she hears the resident talking angrily to himself, but the resident does not answer the nursing assistant. The nursing assistant sees the resident walking around the room and shaking his fist at the air.

Gina: (knock-knock) Mr. Sand? Mr. Sand it's Gina. I've come to help you get ready for breakfast.

Mr. Sand: (to himself) I knew we shouldn't have done it that way! But would they listen to me? Oh no! And now what a mess things are! Well if they think I'm going to fix this they're wrong.

Gina:

Mr. Sand: (to Gina) And you're no better than they are! Who do you think you are coming in here and telling me what to do?

Gina:

Mr. Sand:

_____

Gina:

Nurse:

Gina:

Nurse:

2. A nursing assistant enters a resident's room and correctly identifies himself and the patient. The resident is not happy to see the nursing assistant and begins using bad language and insulting the nursing assistant.

Steven: Good morning, I'm Steven Young, the nursing assistant. Would you like some help getting dressed now Mr.Peterson?

Mr. Peterson: You piece of trash! Get out of here!

Steven:

Mr.Peterson:

Steven:

Nurse:

Steven:

Nurse:

KEEPING THE ENVIRONMENT SAFE

Vocabulary Sentences

1. **Environmental services** should be called to clean up a large spill.
2. Every facility has its own **disaster plan**.

Short Answer

1. List 5 environmental hazards and what to do in each case.

    1. _____

    2. _____

    3. _____

    4. _____

    5. _____

2. List the 5 steps to take if you are trapped by fire.

    1. _____

    2. _____

    3. _____

    4. _____

    5. _____

Writing

Write the words for the following abbreviations. Circle the abbreviations that are the names of diseases.

1. AIDS

_____

2. HIV

_____

3. HBV

_____

4. R-A-C-E

_____

5. OSHA

_____

6. HCV

_____

Listening

Circle the word you hear in each line.

1. incident	intercom	interest
2. splash	sharps	staff
3. document	environment	emergency
4. HIV	HBV	HCV
5. personal	personnel	personally
6. hazard	hazardous	haze

Pronunciation

It can be difficult to hear or pronounce the letters B and V. The B sound is made by putting the lips together but the V sound is made by placing the top front teeth on the bottom lip. Listen and repeat.

1. vase   base
2. vat   bat
3. vile   bile
4. veil   bail
5. veer   beer
6. vend   bend
7. vow   bow
8. HBV
9. HCV
10. HIV
11. violent
12. virus
13. badge
14. body
15. blood

Discussion Questions

1. What should you do if you answer a call light and the patient wants some juice but you have another patient who just asked for help getting to the toilet?

2. What should you do if a patient is smoking in his bed?

3. Explain what the letters R-A-C-E stand for in fire safety.

4. How can you protect yourself from needlesticks and splashes? Why is it important to protect yourself?

LANGUAGE AT WORK

Mrs. Johnson in room 206 rings the call button. The nursing assistant goes to the room immediately.

Darlene:	Mrs. Johnson, how can I help you?
Mrs. Johnson:	Could you please get me some fresh water. My pitcher is empty.
Darlene:	Certainly. I'll get it right away.

Before Darlene can get the water, Mr. Peterson in room 210 rings the call button and Darlene goes into his room.

Darlene:	Yes, Mr. Peterson, what can I do for you?
Mr. Peterson:	I don't feel very well. I'm starting to get some pain in my chest.
Darlene:	OK, Mr. Peterson, I'm going to call the nurse on the intercom and have him check you right away. Stay sitting up in bed and don't try to get up. I'll stay here with you.

The nurse comes in and Darlene reports to him that Mr. Peterson says he is having chest pain. The nurse checks Mr. Peterson and Darlene is asked to bring some equipment to the room.

Darlene returns to Mrs. Johnson's room about 15 minutes later.

Darlene:	Mrs. Johnson, I'm sorry I couldn't get back to you sooner, but we had an emergency. Here's your pitcher of water. Is there anything else you need?
Mrs. Johnson:	Yes, I'd like to know what the emergency was. Did someone die?
Darlene:	I'm sorry. I really can't discuss that with you. Is there something else I can do for you?

Questions

1. Why does Darlene take care of Mr. Peterson before Mrs. Johnson?

_____

2. Why does Darlene stay with Mr. Peterson until the nurse comes?

_____

3. Why doesn't Darlene tell Mrs. Johnson that Mr. Peterson is having chest pain?

_____

COMPETENCY CHECKLIST 1: HEIMLICH MANEUVER

ACTIONS	SATISFACTORY	UNSATISFACTORY (COMMENTS)
Encourage the patient to cough if he can. Call for help and stay with the patient.		
Place thumb side of fist between ribs and navel.		
Push forcefully in and up into the abdomen until food is forced out of airway.		

INSTRUCTOR'S SIGNATURE _____ DATE _____

COMPETENCY CHECKLIST 2: UNCONSCIOUS CHOKING VICTIM

ACTIONS	SATISFACTORY	UNSATISFACTORY (COMMENTS)
With the patient lying on his back, push in and up into the abdomen with the heels of your hands.		
Move to the head and use a finger to remove food.		
Tilt the head and lift the chin.		
Pinch the nose.		
Use mouth shield. Give 2 slow breaths. If the chest does not rise, repeat above actions.		

INSTRUCTOR'S SIGNATURE _____ DATE _____

COMPETENCY CHECKLIST 3: USING GOOD BODY MECHANICS

ACTIONS	SATISFACTORY	UNSATISFACTORY (COMMENTS)
Bend knees and hips. Stand close to object. Keep back straight. Use arm and leg muscles to lift.		
Hold object close to body.		

INSTRUCTOR'S SIGNATURE _____ DATE _____

Chapter 5: Infection Control in the Health Care Institution

VOCABULARY

antibody
autoclave
biohazard
clean utility room
clean
contaminated
diarrhea
dirty utility room
disinfection
disposable
double-bagged
feces
foreign

HIV positive
immune system
infection
infection control
infectious
isolation
lymphatic system
lymphocyte
microbe
mucous membrane
noninfected
nonpathogenic
pathogen

precaution
saliva
semen
sputum
sterile
sterilized
transfusion
universal precautions
urine
vaginal fluid
vomitus
wound drainage
wound

ABBREVIATIONS

AFB   acid-fast bacilli
TB   tuberculosis
PPD   purified protein derivative

MICROBES AND DISEASE

Vocabulary Sentences

1. Most **microbes** are not harmful to people.
2. **Pathogens** are found everywhere.
3. Mr. Smith has an **infection**.
4. Bacteria cause most of the **infectious** diseases people get.
5. **Nonpathogenic** bacteria normally control the amount of yeast in the body.
6. A **mucous membrane** can trap pathogens.
7. HIV causes problems with the **immune system**.
8. The **lymphatic system** extends throughout the body.
9. **Lymphocytes** fight pathogens.
10. **Antibodies** are produced by the blood.

Short Answer

List 6 ways the body protects itself from pathogens.

1. _____

   _____

2. _____

   _____

3. _____

   _____

4. _____

_____

5. _____

_____

6. _____

_____

PREVENTING THE SPREAD OF PATHOGENS

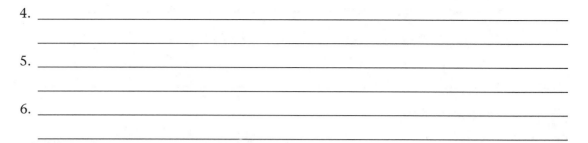

Vocabulary Sentences

1. Pathogens may be spread in **urine**.
2. **Feces** often contain pathogens.
3. **Saliva** of an infected person may contain pathogens.
4. Ms. Jung coughs up a great deal of **sputum**.
5. The emesis basin was full of **vomitus**.
6. **Wound drainage** has soaked the dressing.
7. Pathogens may be spread through **vaginal fluid**.
8. **Semen** can contain pathogens.
9. **Infection control** is one of the most important parts of every health care workers' job.
10. **Universal precautions** must be followed by all health care workers.
11. A patient with HBV may be kept in **isolation**.
12. **Biohazards** must be carefully disposed of.
13. Needles must be **sterile**.
14. Please sterilize these items in the **autoclave**.
15. **Disinfection** is used to clean some medical items.
16. A clean item becomes **contaminated** when it is touched by unwashed hands.
17. Take clean supplies from the **clean utility room**.
18. Bring contaminated supplies to the **dirty utility room**.

Listening

Circle the word you hear in each line.

1. clean	clown	clan
2. faces	feces	focus
3. summon	salmon	semen
4. wand	wound	wind
5. microbe	macro	maker

CONDITIONS AND DISEASES

Vocabulary Sentences

1. A person with HIV is not able to fight off other infections as easily as a **noninfected** person can.
2. When antibodies to HIV are present in a person's blood, the person is **HIV positive**.

Role Play

Choose a nurse, a nursing assistant, and a patient to act out the following scene.

The charge nurse gives the nursing assistant an assignment to take care of a patient with AIDS and TB. The nurse reminds the NA about the precautions she must take to protect herself. The NA takes care of the patient and follows all precautions. Continue the conversation started below and include a conversation between the patient and the NA.

Nurse: Please help Ms. Brooks get ready for bed. She has AIDS and TB so be sure to follow all precautions to protect yourself.

Nursing Assistant: I know how important it is to prevent the spread of pathogens.

Before I go in her room I'll _____.

I also need to _____

_____

_____.

Nurse: That's right. And please remember to _____.

Report back to me when you are finished.

Nursing Assistant:

_____

(The nursing assistant acts out the precautions she should take before entering the room.)

Nursing Assistant:

Ms. Brooks:

Nursing Assistant:

Ms. Brooks:

(Continue this conversation to an ending. You may also wish to have the nursing assistant report back to the nurse.)

Crossword Puzzle

Write the correct word in the spaces, Figure 5–1.

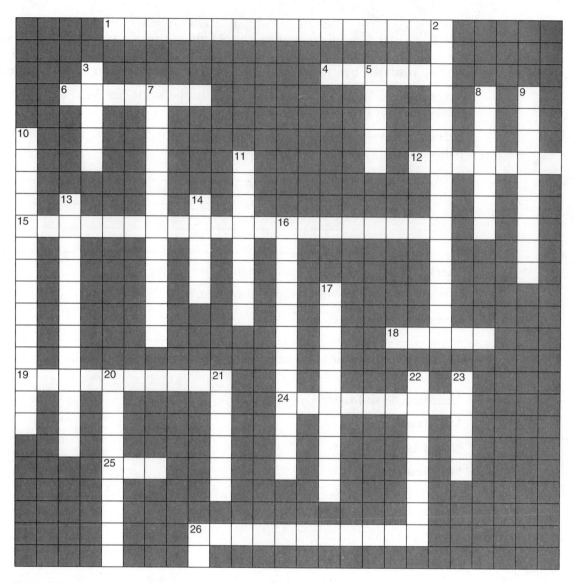

Figure 5–1

Across
1. Prevention of the spread of infection from one person to another
4. A substance that comes from the lungs and breathing passages that is coughed up and spit out of the mouth
6. Becoming dirty
12. No microbes are present
15. The set of rules to prevent the spread of diseases caused by blood-borne pathogens
18. Fluid containing sperm that is made by the reproductive organs of a man
19. Substances produced by the blood to fight pathogens
24. Machine that sterilizes items using steam under pressure
25. Abbreviation for acid-fast bacilli
26. Blood is taken from one person, processed at a laboratory, and given to another person

Down

2. Collects extra body fluid from the blood, cleans it, and returns it to the blood; also produces lymphocytes
3. Open area on the skin
5. The liquid waste that comes out of the body
7. The system of the body that fights pathogens
8. A tiny living organism that can only be seen with a microscope
9. The patient and everything used by the patient is kept separate from other patients
10. The lining inside passages of the body which make a fluid called mucous
11. Many watery bowel movements
13. A cleaning process that kills pathogens
14. Free of pathogens
16. Dirty; pathogens are present
17. Easily spread from one person to another; contagious, communicable
20. Any material contaminated with blood or body fluids that may be infectious
21. The liquid that is made by the salivary glands in the mouth
22. A microbe that causes disease
23. The solid waste that passes out of the body
26. Abbreviation for tuberculosis

What Would You Say?

1. What could you say to a patient who asks you, "Why are you wearing gloves? I don't have AIDS!"

2. What could you say to a co-worker who does not wear gloves when handling body fluids?

3. A patient asks you "Aren't you afraid you'll catch AIDS working as a nursing assistant?" Explain to this patient how AIDS is spread and what precautions you take to protect yourself.

LANGUAGE AT WORK

Massoud: I can't believe how many times I washed my hands today, Kim.

Kim: Me too, Massoud. We've been so busy I must have washed my hands 50 times! Sometimes I get tired of it but I know it's the most important way to prevent diseases from spreading.

Massoud: You're right about that. But sometimes handwashing isn't enough. I'm glad they have boxes of disposable gloves in every room.

Kim: Today I also have a patient in AFB isolation. It's difficult working with that mask on. But it's even worse for my patient. She gets very sad when she sees that even her family has to wear masks when they come to see her. I try to encourage her as much as I can to continue with the treatment her doctor has ordered.

Massoud: Well, I'd better finish up with my work. See you later.

Questions

1. What has Kim had to do many times today?

_____

2. What else does Massoud do to practice infection control?

_____

3. What disease does the patient in AFB isolation have?

_____

4. Why does the patient become sad?

_____

5. How can the nursing assistant help the patient who is in isolation?

_____

COMPETENCY CHECKLIST 4: HANDWASHING

ACTIONS	SATISFACTORY	UNSATISFACTORY (COMMENTS)
Adjust water to warm temperature.		
Wet hands, let water flow downward.		
Apply soap.		
Rub hands together up to wrists.		
Rub nails against palms.		
Rinse, let water flow downward.		
Dry hands with paper towel.		
Turn off faucets with another paper towel.		
Apply lotion to hands, if needed.		

INSTRUCTOR'S SIGNATURE _____ DATE _____

COMPETENCY CHECKLIST 5: USING GLOVES

ACTIONS	SATISFACTORY	UNSATISFACTORY (COMMENTS)
Wash hands if necessary, put on correct size gloves.		
Grasp one glove at the palm.		
Pull glove off.		
Hold the removed glove in the gloved hand.		
Use 2 or 3 fingers of ungloved hand under edge of other glove and pull off inside out.		
Dispose of gloves in trash container.		
Wash hands.		

INSTRUCTOR'S SIGNATURE _____ DATE _____

COMPETENCY CHECKLIST 6: UNIVERSAL PRECAUTIONS

ACTIONS	SATISFACTORY	UNSATISFACTORY (COMMENTS)
Use gloves when touching blood and body fluids.		
Wash hands after removing gloves. Wash immediately any contaminated part of body.		
Use eyewear, face shields and gowns for possible splashes.		
Dispose of sharps in sharps containers.		
Use resuscitation mouthpiece or bag.		
Use special containers for contaminated trash and linen.		

INSTRUCTOR'S SIGNATURE _____ DATE _____

COMPETENCY CHECKLIST 7: ISOLATION PRECAUTIONS

ACTIONS	SATISFACTORY	UNSATISFACTORY (COMMENTS)
Take off gloves.		
Untie waist strings.		
Remove mask.		
Untie neck strings.		
Cross arms and grasp neck strings.		
Using ties, pull off gown inside out.		
Remove gown and roll into a ball, holding it away from you.		
Wash hands.		

INSTRUCTOR'S SIGNATURE _____ DATE _____

Chapter 6: Human Growth and Development

VOCABULARY

aging
agitated
Alzheimer's disease
bedpan
career
congenital
couple
dementia
dependent
development
dim
disoriented
eliminate
emotional
fantasy
growth spurt
hard of hearing

independence
infant
loses balance
masturbate
menopause
mentally retarded
mood
newborn
peer pressure
perspiration
physical
process
psychologist
psychotherapy
reality orientation
reality
reminisce

restraint
retirement
rule out
self-esteem
senior citizen
social
spouse
stress
suicide
sundowning
teenager
terminal
triple
unique
urinal
validation therapy
wander

ABBREVIATIONS

HOH   hard of hearing

DEVELOPMENTAL AGES AND STAGES

Vocabulary Sentences

1. Teenagers are under a great deal of **peer pressure**.
2. **Self-esteem** is a basic need for all people.
3. **Menopause** can be a difficult time for women.
4. As people age they may become **hard of hearing**.
5. Some older people become **dependent** on others for their care.
6. Having **stress** in your life can cause you to have health problems.

Culture Exchange

In the text we discussed what it is like to be a teenager in the United States. What is life like for a teenager in your country? Answer the following questions alone or with class-mates from your country. Then share your answers with the rest of the class.

1. What do adolescents in your country do with their time? Do they work? go to school? get married and have children?

_____

_____

_____

2. What is the normal relationship between an adolescent and his parents?

_____

_____

_____

3. What is the normal relationship between middle-aged adults and their elderly parents?

_____

_____

_____

4. What is thought to be a good age for women to have children in your country? What age is too young to have children?

_____

_____

_____

5. What makes a person an adult in your country? Is there a special age when a child becomes an adult?

_____

_____

_____

6. How are elderly people treated in your birth country?

_____

_____

_____

BASIC HUMAN NEEDS

Vocabulary Sentences

1. **Perspiration** is one way the body **eliminates** wastes.
2. A **urinal** allows men to urinate without going to the toilet.
3. Mr. Hall is on the **bedpan** right now.
4. Are **spouses** invited to the holiday party?

Short Answer

List 6 physical needs. For each need give 1 way a nursing assistant could help a patient meet that need.

1. _____

_____

2. _____

_____

3. _____

_____

4. _____

_____

5. _____

_____

6. _____

List 5 emotional needs. For each need give 1 way a nursing assistant could help a patient meet that need.

1. _____

_____

2. _____

_____

3. _____

_____

4. _____

_____

5. _____

_____

Grammar

Underline the word "need" in each of the following sentences. You will see it with different endings. For each sentence, tell whether the word "need" is used as noun or a verb. Examples:

_____noun_____1. Patients have many different <u>needs</u>.

_____verb_____2. He <u>needs</u> breakfast.

_____3. I need something to drink.

_____4. What do you need?

_____5. A nursing assistant helps meet the needs of the patient.

_____6. Everyone needs to feel loved.

_____7. Self-esteem is an important emotional need.

_____8. She needed some rest.

_____9. Our basic needs can be met in many different ways.

MASLOW'S HIERARCHY OF NEEDS

Vocabulary Sentences

1. Abraham Maslow was a famous **psychologist**.

Listening

Listen to your instructor read each of the following sentences. When you hear something different from what is written, circle it and write the new word on the line before the sentence.

_____1. A nursing assistant can help a patient sleep by making the room bright and quiet.

_____2. The dietitian helps patients meet their need for food and intimacy.

_____ 3. You cannot meet a patient's need for sexual intimacy, but you can give him the activity he needs by always knocking before opening doors and speaking before opening curtains.

_____ 4. Emotional needs are harder to give care of than physical needs.

_____ 5. Encouraging a patient to be as independent as possible helps him find his need for self-esteem.

_____ 6. Some elderly people live on skilled nursing facilities.

_____ 7. During the growing process the human body and mind both slow down.

_____ 8. Even at age 85 or younger, some people are still able to live independently.

_____ 9. Self-actualization is the first step in Maslow's hierarchy of needs.

_____10. Health care workers must always make respect for the patient.

CONDITIONS AND DISEASES

Vocabulary Sentences

1. Mental retardation is often a **congenital** disease.
2. A person with a psychological disorder may be helped with **psychotherapy**.
3. Some people have trouble telling the difference between **reality** and **fantasy**.
4. We cannot **rule out** loneliness as a cause of her depression.
5. Door alarms help keep residents who **wander** safe.
6. Michael just found out he has a **terminal** disease.
7. Senior citizens often like to **reminisce**.
8. Mr. Appleby was very **agitated** this morning.

Pronunciation

In this exercise, the letter 'o' is pronounced in 2 ways. 'O' may sound like 'o' as in coat or 'o' as in cover. Listen to the pronunciation of the following words as you read the word in your workbook. Stop the tape after each word and write the word in the correct column.

psychotherapy   emotional   congenital
couple   menopause   social
process   growth spurt   hard of hearing
development

'o' as in coat   'o' as in cover

_____   _____

_____   _____

_____   _____

_____   _____

_____   _____

_____   _____

What Do You Say?

Below are several situations involving patients with dementia. For each situation write a correct response for a nursing assistant to make based on what you learned in this chapter.

1. While drinking a glass of juice, a patient suddenly forgets what she is doing. She pours the juice all over her shirt and the table.
Correct Response:

_____

_____

2. On a cold winter morning a resident comes to breakfast wearing shorts and sandals.
Correct Response:

_____

_____

3. When you greet a patient in the morning he tells you, "Get down! Do you want them to see you? You'll be shot!" He thinks he is in the middle of a war.
Correct Response:

_____

_____

Role Play

Choose 1 student to play the nursing assistant and another to play the patient. Begin the scene when the nursing assistant enters the room.

A patient with dementia is found sitting on the floor of his room with wet pants. When the nursing assistant comes in he looks at her like he doesn't know her and acts afraid. He begins talking about the beach and asks where the children are.

Patient: I want to go to the beach, too. Where did the other children go?

NA:

Patient:

(Continue the conversation. Try to end the conversation with the nursing assistant helping the patient change into other clothes to go to the dining room for lunch.)

Discussion Question

1. What are some things a nursing assistant can do to help a patient with dementia? What are some things a facility can do to help a patient with dementia?

LANGUAGE AT WORK

The nursing assistant talks with Mrs. Anderson, the daughter of an elderly patient on the medical-surgical floor of a general hospital.

Silva: Hello, Mrs. Anderson. Did you have a good visit with your father today?

Mrs. Anderson: He seemed happy to see me, but was disoriented about where he is. It makes me worry that he won't be able to live with me anymore.

Silva: You sound concerned about where your father should live when he leaves the hospital.

Mrs. Anderson: I am. I don't know if it is better to have him live in a nursing home or live with me and my family. I worry that he won't be able to stay alone while my husband and I are at work. But maybe he will feel that I don't love him if I place him in a nursing home.

Silva: That's a difficult decision to make. Your father could be well cared for in a nursing home. But maybe you'd rather have him at home?

Mrs. Anderson: I do like having him there and it's good for my children to know their grandfather.

Silva: Do you know that there is adult day care at the senior center? He can do activities and spend time with people his age during the day when you're at work. I can ask the nurse to speak to you about it.

Mrs. Anderson: That sounds like a great idea. I'd like to find out more about it. Then I'll ask my father what he thinks about it. Thanks for your help!

Questions

1. Who is Mrs. Anderson visiting in the hospital?

_____

2. Why is Mrs. Anderson worried?

_____

3. Why does Mrs. Anderson like having her father at home?

_____

4. What suggestion does Silva make to Mrs. Anderson?

_____

5. What does Mrs. Anderson plan to do now?

_____

Chapter 7: Communications in the Health Care Setting

VOCABULARY

blind
body language
communication
deaf
gestures
interpreter

negative attitude
nonverbal
opinion
prejudge
prejudice

pretend
read lips
upset
verbal
worry

COMMUNICATION BASICS

Vocabulary Sentences

1. We use **communication** skills to let other people know what we are thinking.
2. We use **verbal** communication when we speak on the telephone.
3. Smiling is an example of **nonverbal** communication.
4. **Gestures** can have different meanings in different cultures.
5. **Body language** can communicate that we are interested in what someone is saying to us.

Short Answer

Give 2 examples of verbal communication.

1. _____

2. _____

Give 2 examples of nonverbal communication.

1. _____

2. _____

COMMUNICATING WITH STAFF, PATIENTS, AND VISITORS

Vocabulary Sentences

1. Patients in the hospital often have many **worries**.
2. Nursing assistants do not need to share their **opinions** with the patients.
3. Mr. Sanelli was **upset** after he spoke to the doctor.

What Do You Say?

Imagine that a patient said the following things to you. Write a good response to each sentence on the line below the sentence. Remember that is not your job to give your opinion or to solve the patient's problems. Your job is to listen and encourage the patient to talk about what is bothering him.

1. I can't stand to stay in this hospital anymore!

_____

_____

_____

2. What do you think happens after you die?

_____

_____

_____

3. The doctor says I'll get better, but I don't believe it. I think they are just saying that, but they know I will die soon.

_____

_____

_____

4. I used to go to church but I haven't gone for a long time. I guess God has forgotten me by now.

_____

_____

_____

5. I'm no longer important to anyone.

_____

_____

_____

6. I've got to get well. My wife and kids can't manage without me.

_____

_____

_____

7. Do you like that nurse?

_____

_____

_____

8. I don't know if I should have this surgery.

_____

_____

_____

Role Play

Choose a student to play the role of nursing assistant and another to play the role of the patient. If needed, you may choose a nurse as well.

Nursing Assistant: Good morning! How are you feeling this morning?

Patient: What difference does it make? I'm going to die soon anyway.

(Continue this conversation with at least one more response by the nursing assistant and the patient.)

IMPROVING COMMUNICATION

Vocabulary Sentences

1. Health care workers must not **pretend** to understand instructions.

Short Answer

You are a nursing assistant in a hospital. You have been asked to take a patient from her room to radiology. What 6 things do you need to do to make sure you send a clear message to the patient?

1. _____

_____

2. _____

_____

3. _____

_____

4. _____

_____

5. _____

_____

6. _____

_____

If the patient does not understand you, what 3 things can you try to help her understand?

1. _____

2. _____

3. _____

You are a nursing assistant in a long-term care facility. You are filling water pitchers when the nurse comes up to talk to you. List 5 things you should do to be a good listener in this situation.

1. _____

_____

2. _____

_____

3. _____

_____

4. _____

_____

5. _____

_____

BARRIERS TO CLEAR COMMUNICATION

Vocabulary Sentences

1. Many health care facilities have **interpreters** to help patients who speak a different language.
2. A patient who is **deaf** needs special help communicating.
3. Some deaf people know how to **read lips**.
4. Although **blind** patients can hear, you may still need to use special methods of communication.
5. A **negative attitude** can be a big problem in communications.
6. **Prejudice** is often a bigger barrier to communication than deafness or blindness.
7. People should be treated as individuals and not be **prejudged**.

Listening

Listen and circle the word you hear in each line.

1. blind	bind	bland
2. prejudge	prejudice	pretend
3. theft	deaf	left
4. interpreter	intensive	intercom
5. hurry	curry	worry

Writing

Write a paragraph explaining how prejudice has made clear communication difficult in your life. It may be a story about when you prejudged someone and then found out you were wrong or about a time when someone prejudged you.

_____

_____

_____

_____

_____

_____

Discussion Question

1. Why is good communication so important in a health care facility?

LANGUAGE AT WORK

Nursing assistants who work on the same floor are discussing a resident of a nursing home. Both of these nursing assistants take care of Mr. Sheehan on different days. Today Kathy was told by the nurse to give him a bath.

Kathy: Mr. Sheehan is so confused today. He didn't understand when I explained that I wanted to help him with his bath this morning.

Mary: I know. Yesterday his daughter came to visit him and he didn't know who she was.

Kathy: Sometimes he says a few words to me and smiles, but this morning he was very sad. I was so surprised when he started to cry.

Mary: What did you do?

Kathy: I didn't know what to do at first. I asked him if he could tell me what was making him cry, but he didn't answer me. I decided to cover him, raise the side-rail and ask the nurse what I should do.

Mary: Did she want you to continue with the bath?

Kathy: No, she said that it wasn't important to give him the bath now. Perhaps I can do it after he eats his breakfast.

Mary: Maybe I'll go in and see him for a little while. Even though he has Alzheimer's disease, he sometimes talks to me about the flower garden he had years ago. He seems to remember the names of flowers, even though he can't always remember his own name. Maybe that will put him in a better mood. Then you can try helping him with his bath later.

Questions

1. What does "confused" mean?

   _____

2. What should you do if a patient says that he doesn't want you to touch him?

   _____

3. What did Kathy remember to do before leaving Mr. Sheehan's bedside to talk to the nurse?

   _____

4. What is Alzheimer's disease?

   _____

5. What does Mr. Sheehan like to reminisce about?

   _____

Chapter 8: Clerical Communication

VOCABULARY

allergy
alphabetize
ambulatory
cheerful
cooperative
forgetful

last name
mental attitude
nicknames
orientation
prefix

scalp
sharp
uncooperative
urgent
valuables

ABBREVIATIONS

NKA no known allergies
NKDA no known drug allergies

ANSWERING THE TELEPHONE

Vocabulary Sentences

1. American **last names** come from all over the world.
2. Please give him this message right away, it's **urgent**.

Short Answer

Complete the conversation with what you would say if you were a nursing assistant answering the phone at the Pine Street Clinic. Start from when you first pick up the phone.

A. _____

B. I'd like to speak to Dr. White, please.

A. _____

B. This is Kelly Brandt.

A. _____

B. K-E-L-L-Y B-R-A-N-D-T

A. _____

B. Well, I have a pain in my ear and I cannot hear well.

A. _____

B. 555-2343

A. _____

B. That's right.

A. _____

B. Anytime after 2:00.

A. _____

B. Thank you.

A. _____

B. Good-bye.

Now fill out the message form for this conversation on the form below, Figure 8–1.

```
┌─────────────────────────────────────────┐
│         ╭─────────────────────╮          │
│         │      MESSAGE         │          │
│         ╰─────────────────────╯          │
│  FOR _____    │
│                                  A.M.     │
│  DATE _____ TIME _____ P.M.     │
│  M _____│
│  OF _____│
│  PHONE _____│
│        AREA CODE    NUMBER    EXTENSION   │
│  ┌──────────────────┬┬─────────────────┬┐│
│  │ TELEPHONED       ││ PLEASE CALL     ││ │
│  ├──────────────────┼┼─────────────────┼┤│
│  │ WANTS TO SEE YOU ││ URGENT          ││ │
│  ├──────────────────┼┼─────────────────┼┤│
│  │ RETURNED YOUR CALL││ WILL CALL AGAIN ││ │
│  └──────────────────┴┴─────────────────┴┘│
│                                           │
│  MESSAGE _____ │
│  _____│
│  _____│
│  _____│
│  _____│
│                                           │
│  SIGNED _____ │
└─────────────────────────────────────────┘
```

Figure 8–1

Writing

Follow the instructions for answering telephones to write your own telephone conversation. You may use the phrases listed in the textbook or make up your own. Your conversation should have 2 people, with each saying at least 10 things.

A. _____

B. _____

A. _____

B. _____

A. _____

B. _____

A. _____

B. _____

A. _____

B. _____

A. _____

B. _____

A. _____

B. _____

A. _____

B. _____

A. _____

B. _____

A. _____

B. _____

FILING

Vocabulary Sentences

1. When filing we put names in **alphabetical** order.

Short Answer

Indexing Names.   Put the following names into indexing order—last name, first name, middle name. Remember to watch out for 2-part last names!

1. Jill St. James

   _____

2. Susan L. DeBell

   _____

3. Dana Lynne Smith

   _____

4. John Van Johnson

   _____

5. Jack William Jones

   _____

6. Emily DiPaola

   _____

7. John Robert Thompson

   _____

8. Carl B. Miller

   _____

9. Carmen L. Martinez

   _____

10. Fred P. McIntyre

    _____

11. Zhe Hua Chen

    _____

12. John K. Ellis

    _____

13. Vicki White

_____

14. Joao Gomes

_____

15. Tony La Rocco

_____

16. Mary Sue Snow

_____

17. Walter F. O'Reilley

_____

18. Luzia Andrade

_____

19. Maria DelMonte

_____

20. Glenn D'Arby

_____

Filing.   Put the names below in indexing order, then put the list in alphabetical order.

Name	Indexing Order
Richard Shiff	_____
H. L. Sheridan	_____
Emma Marie Shield	_____
Arthur J. Sherman	_____
Henry A. Sherr	_____

Alphabetical Order

_____

_____

_____

_____

_____

Name	Indexing Order
Devin Del Monte	_____
Sally Davison	_____
David D'Abate	_____
Daniel Peter Davis	_____
Karen D. Dacus	_____
Corine De Fusco	_____
Kelly L. Dagg	_____

Alphabetical Order

_____

_____

_____

_____

_____

_____

_____

A B C D E F G H I J K L M N O P Q R S T U V W X Y Z

ADMISSIONS

Vocabulary Sentences

1. Mr. Roshkam is an **ambulatory** patient.
2. Betty is a **nickname** for Elizabeth.
3. **Orientation** is a good way to learn about a new place.
4. Always know where your **valuables** are.
5. Regular hair washing helps keep the **scalp** clean.
6. A patient's **mental attitude** affects how she feels physically.
7. An **uncooperative** patient can be difficult to care for.
8. **Cooperative** nursing assistants are a pleasure to work with.
9. Mr. Giese is always so **cheerful**.
10. Patients with Alzheimer's disease are often **forgetful**.
11. Even though her body is weak, Mrs. DeBell's mind is **sharp**.

Matching

Match the words in the left column to their descriptions in the right column.

___1. allergies

___2. likes to be called

___3. medical aids

___4. mode of transportation

___5. orientation

___6. speaks English minimally

___7. valuables

___8. vital signs

a. clothing, jewelry, or money
b. dentures, glasses or contacts, or hearing aids
c. does not speak English well
d. name a patient wishes to be called
e. showing a patient where things are and how they work
f. temperature, pulse, respirations, and blood pressure
g. wheelchair, ambulatory, or stretcher
h. unusual reaction to medication or food

Short Answer

Write the opposite for each of the words below.

1. formal _____

2. cooperative _____

3. oriented _____

4. forgetful _____

LANGUAGE AT WORK

In the following conversations nursing assistants are answering the telephone while at work. Note how the conversations are the same and how they are different.

Conversation #1

Mrs. Martinez:	Good morning, Women's Health Center, Mrs. Martinez, Nursing Assistant speaking. May I help you?
Maria LeSage:	Good morning. May I speak with Mr. LeSage, please?
Mrs. Martinez:	May I ask who is calling?
Maria LeSage:	This is his daughter, Maria.
Mrs. Martinez:	One moment, please.

Conversation #2

Mr. Chin:	Good afternoon, Dr. Po's office, Mr. Chin, Nursing Assistant speaking. May I help you?
Veronica Gomes:	I'd like to speak to the doctor, please.
Mr. Chin:	May I ask who is calling?
Veronica Gomes:	This is Veronica Gomes.
Mr. Chin:	Ms. Gomes, the doctor isn't in right now, may I take a message?
Veronica Gomes:	No, I'll call back later.
Mr. Chin:	Thank you for calling. Good-bye.
Veronica Gomes:	Good-bye.

Conversation #3

Ms. Sanelli:	Good morning, Maternity Department, Ms. Sanelli, CNA speaking. May I help you?
Linda Kingsley:	Yes, I'm trying to reach Susan McMann.
Ms. Sanelli:	I'm sorry, Susan is with a patient right now. May I take a message?
Linda Kingsley:	Yes. Please tell her I called.
Ms. Sanelli:	May I have your name please?
Linda Kingsley:	Linda Kingsley.
Ms. Sanelli:	Would you spell that for me?
Linda Kingsley:	L-i-n-d-a, K-i-n-g-s-l-e-y.
Ms. Sanelli:	L-i-n-d-a, K-i-n-g-s-l-e-y?
Linda Kingsley:	That's right.
Ms. Sanelli:	Any message?
Linda Kingsley:	I'm calling from Dr. Frank's office. Please have her call me.
Ms. Sanelli:	Your telephone number, please?
Linda Kingsley:	(807) 555-8980.
Ms. Sanelli:	(807) 555-8980?
Linda Kingsley:	Yes.
Ms. Sanelli:	When is the best time for her to reach you?
Linda Kingsley:	I'll be here until 1:00 this afternoon.
Ms. Sanelli:	I'll give Susan your message.
Linda Kingsley:	Thank you. Good-bye.
Ms. Sanelli:	Good-bye.

Questions

1. The nursing assistant in conversation #2 says "Ms. Gomes," using the title and the last name. The nursing assistant in conversation #3 says simply, "Susan." Why do you think there is this difference?

   _____

2. Fill out a message form based on conversation #3, Figure 8–2. Use today's date and time.

```
╭─────────────────────────────────────────╮
│        ╭──────────────────────╮         │
│        │      MESSAGE         │         │
│        ╰──────────────────────╯         │
│  FOR _____   │
│                                   A.M.   │
│  DATE _____ TIME _____  P.M.   │
│  M _____   │
│  OF _____   │
│  PHONE _____   │
│        AREA CODE   NUMBER   EXTENSION    │
│  ┌─────────────────┬┬──────────────┬┐   │
│  │ TELEPHONED      ││ PLEASE CALL  ││   │
│  │ WANTS TO SEE YOU││ URGENT       ││   │
│  │ RETURNED YOUR CALL││ WILL CALL AGAIN││ │
│  └─────────────────┴┴──────────────┴┘   │
│  MESSAGE _____   │
│  _____   │
│  _____   │
│  _____   │
│  _____   │
│  SIGNED _____   │
╰─────────────────────────────────────────╯
```

Figure 8–2

Chapter 9: Using Medical Terminology to Observe and Describe the Patient

VOCABULARY

abbreviation	lateral	prefix
acronym	medial	quadrant
anterior	medical terminology	restless
cell	noisy	state
complain of	observation	suffix
dorsal	opinion	tissue
epigastric	organ	umbilicus
fact	planes	ventral
foul	posterior	word root

ABBREVIATIONS

c/o   complains of
L   left
LLQ   left lower quadrant
LUQ   left upper quadrant

R   right
RLQ   right lower quadrant
RUQ   right upper quadrant

MEDICAL TERMINOLOGY

Vocabulary Sentences

1. Health care workers find their jobs much easier when they understand **medical terminology**.
2. Knowing **word roots** helps you figure out word meanings.
3. Many **suffixes** and **prefixes** used in medical terminology are used throughout the English language.

Short Answer

Divide the following words into word roots, suffixes, and prefixes. Label each part with its meaning.

Example: dyspnea   dys = difficult   pnea = breathing

1. cardiology _____

2. apnea _____

3. audiologist _____

4. cardiovascular _____

5. nasogastric _____

6. gastritis _____

7. psychologist _____

8. neurology _____

9. hypotension _____

10. bradycardia _____

ABBREVIATIONS

Vocabulary Sentences

1. Medical **abbreviations** make communicating in the health care setting faster and easier.

Writing

Write 5 sentences using abbreviations from Chapters 1 through 9. Use at least 2 abbreviations in each sentence.

1. _____
2. _____
3. _____
4. _____
5. _____

DESCRIBING THE HUMAN BODY

Vocabulary Sentences

1. Many different kinds of **cells** work together to make the human body.
2. Different **tissues** perform different functions in the body.
3. The heart, liver, and stomach are examples of **organs**.
4. The patient has a red area on the **anterior** part of his upper thigh.
5. The patient complains of pain in the **ventral** right upper quadrant.
6. We sit on the lower **posterior** part of our bodies.
7. Nursing assistants must watch for red areas on the **dorsal** plane of patients who must stay in bed.
8. Mr. Jenkins has a wound on the left lower quadrant in the **lateral** plane.
9. The **umbilicus** is at the center of the 4 **quadrants** of the abdomen.
10. The patient complains of pain in the **epigastric** area after eating.

Describe the Place on the Body

Write the numbers 1, 2, 3, 4, 5, and 6 on different places on Figure 9–1. Then describe the places on the body on the lines below using the medical words you have learned in this chapter.

1. _____
2. _____
3. _____
4. _____
5. _____
6. _____

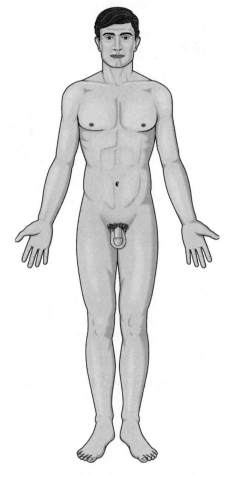

Figure 9–1

Short Answer

Write the opposite of each word or word part listed below.

1. right _____

2. anterior _____

3. dorsal _____

4. upper _____

5. pre _____

6. hyper _____

7. brady _____

OBSERVING THE PATIENT

Vocabulary Sentence

1. When a nursing assistant makes **observations** about the patient, it gives the nurse important information.

Writing

Look at Figure 9–8 in the text book. List 3 opinions and 3 facts about the patient. Make some different observations from those given in the textbook.

Opinion

1. _____

2. _____

3. _____

Fact

1. _____

2. _____

3. _____

Fact or Opinion

Decide if each of the observations below is a fact or an opinion. If it is a fact, write FACT in the space. If it is an opinion, write OPINION in the space.

_____ 1. The patient seems tired.

_____ 2. The patient is asleep.

_____ 3. I think the patient needs another blanket.

_____ 4. The patient must feel nauseous.

_____ 5. The patient refused to eat her lunch.

_____ 6. The patient has a red area on the anterior lower right leg.

_____ 7. The bandage on the patient's right hand has blood on it.

_____ 8. The patient states "I have a lot of pain in my stomach."

_____ 9. I think the patient got up during the night to urinate.

_____10. It seems like the patient has pain in his left upper quadrant.

Discussion Questions

1. What kinds of things might a nursing assistant report to her supervisor? Why are her observations so important?

2. What is medical jargon and why is it used?

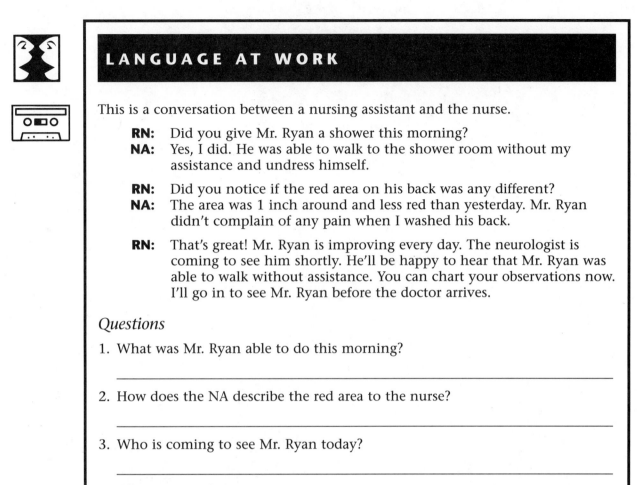

LANGUAGE AT WORK

This is a conversation between a nursing assistant and the nurse.

RN: Did you give Mr. Ryan a shower this morning?

NA: Yes, I did. He was able to walk to the shower room without my assistance and undress himself.

RN: Did you notice if the red area on his back was any different?

NA: The area was 1 inch around and less red than yesterday. Mr. Ryan didn't complain of any pain when I washed his back.

RN: That's great! Mr. Ryan is improving every day. The neurologist is coming to see him shortly. He'll be happy to hear that Mr. Ryan was able to walk without assistance. You can chart your observations now. I'll go in to see Mr. Ryan before the doctor arrives.

Questions

1. What was Mr. Ryan able to do this morning?

   _____

2. How does the NA describe the red area to the nurse?

   _____

3. Who is coming to see Mr. Ryan today?

   _____

4. Where will the NA chart her observations?

   _____

Chapter 10: Respiratory System and Cardiovascular System/Taking Vital Signs

VOCABULARY

accurately
alcohol prep
alveoli
angina
aorta
apical pulse
artery
asthma
atherosclerosis
atria
aural
axillary
blood pressure
blood vessel
brachial
bradycardia
bronchi
bronchioles
capillary
carbon dioxide
cardiac arrest
cardiovascular system
carotid
cerebrovascular
    accident
chart
chills
chronic obstructive
    pulmonary disease
circulate
circulatory system
congestive heart failure

contract
coronary artery disease
coronary
cyanosis
deflate
diaphragm
diastolic
dilate
dyspnea
electrocardiogram
embolism
emphysema
exchange of gases
exhalation
expiration
femoral
fever
flow chart
flowmeter
graphic chart
hypertension
hypotension
inflate
inhalation
inspiration
irritation
larynx
lubricant
mercury
myocardial infarction
nasal cavity
normal range

nostril
oral cavity
oxygen
pallor
pedal
pharynx
pneumonia
productive cough
pulmonary edema
pulse
radial
rectal
respiration
shortness of breath
sign
strep throat
sweats
symptom
systolic
tachycardia
temperature
thermometer
thrombophlebitis
thrombus
trachea
tympanic
vein
vena cava
ventricle
vital signs
waste product
wheezing

ABBREVIATIONS

@	at	**EKG** or **ECG**	electrocardiogram
AP	apical	**F**	Fahrenheit
AX	axillary	**HTN**	hypertension
BP	blood pressure	**irr**	irregular
C	Celsius	**L**	liter
CAD	coronary artery disease	**MI**	myocardial infarction
CHF	congestive heart failure	**min**	minute
CO2	carbon dioxide	**NC**	nasal canula
COPD	chronic obstructive pulmonary disease	**O2**	oxygen
		°	degrees
CVA	cerebrovascular accident	**P**	pulse

R	respiration	**sx**	symptoms
R	rectal	**T**	temperature
SOB	shortness of breath	**URI**	upper respiratory infection
stat	immediately	**VS**	vital signs

HOW THE RESPIRATORY SYSTEM AND THE CARDIOVASCULAR SYSTEM WORK TOGETHER

Vocabulary Sentences

1. We breathe in **oxygen**, which is needed by body cells.
2. **Carbon dioxide** is produced as a waste product by the cells.
3. When I have a cold my **nasal cavity** has mucous in it.
4. Dentists take care of many problems in the **oral cavity**
5. The air we breathe travels through the **pharynx**.
6. The **trachea** is often called the windpipe.
7. An inflammation of the **bronchi** is called bronchitis.
8. When we breathe in, our **lungs** fill with air.
9. The **capillaries** have very thin walls.
10. The **exchange of gases** occurs in the lungs.
11. **Inspiration** and **inhalation** bring oxygen into our bodies.
12. **Expiration** and **exhalation** take carbon dioxide out of our bodies.
13. There are many **blood vessels** all through our bodies.
14. **Arteries** and **veins** are part of the cardiovascular system.
15. The **aorta** comes out of the left **ventricle**.
16. The **vena cava** brings blood to the right atrium.
17. The heart contains 2 **atria** and 2 **ventricles**.
18. The **circulatory system** allows blood to travel to every cell of the body.

Label the Diagrams

Label the parts of the respiratory system, Figure 10–1.

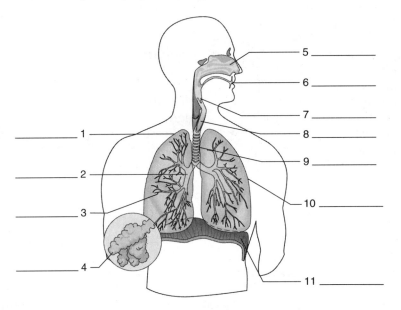

Figure 10–1

Label the parts of the cardiovascular system, Figure 10–2.

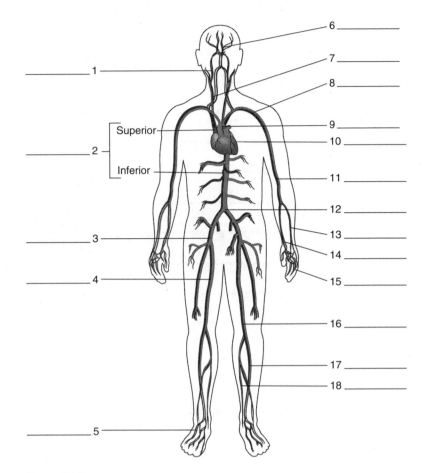

Figure 10–2

VITAL SIGNS

Vocabulary Sentences

1. The nursing assistant may be responsible for taking vital signs on patients.
2. The 4 vital signs are **temperature, pulse, respiration,** and **blood pressure**.
3. If the patient has a **fever** the nurse must be informed **stat**.
4. You must shake down the **mercury** in a glass **thermometer** before using it.
5. The **axillary** method of taking the temperature is the least accurate.
6. The **rectal** method of taking the temperature is often used with small children who might bite a glass thermometer.
7. The **tympanic** method of taking the temperature is the newest and fastest.
8. Mrs. Long's **apical pulse** is 72.
9. Mr. Chan had **cyanosis** around his mouth.
10. If **bradycardia** or **tachycardia** is unusual for a patient, the nursing assistant must report it to the nurse stat.
11. When taking the respirations, a nursing assistant must report any **dyspnea** or **SOB**.
12. Blood pressure is expressed as the **systolic** number over the **diastolic** number.
13. You must carefully pronounce **hypertension** and **hypotension** to avoid confusion.
14. A **graphic chart** allows us to see a picture of the patient's vital signs over a period of several days.
15. The **radial pulse** is located at the wrist, on the thumb side.

Short Answer

1. Read the following thermometers and write the temperature in the space provided. Be sure to write "F" for Fahrenheit and "C" for Celsius, Figure 10–3.

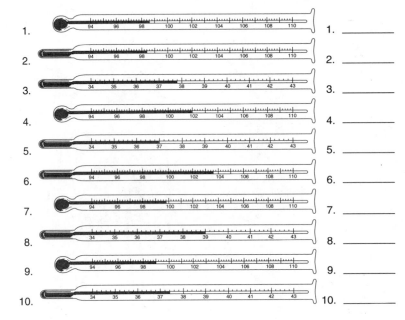

1. 1. _____
2. 2. _____
3. 3. _____
4. 4. _____
5. 5. _____
6. 6. _____
7. 7. _____
8. 8. _____
9. 9. _____
10. 10. _____

Figure 10–3

2. Read the following blood pressure dials and write the number that the pointer is at in the space provided, Figure 10–4.

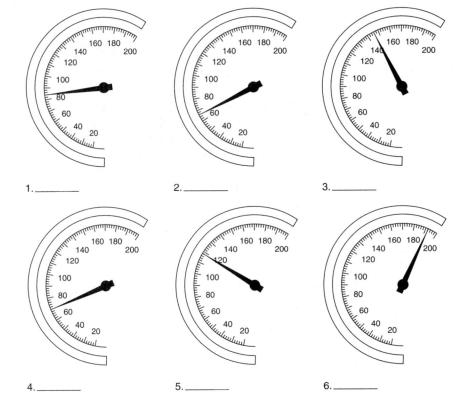

1. _____   2. _____   3. _____

4. _____   5. _____   6. _____

Figure 10–4

3. Read the following columns of mercury and write the number in the space provided, Figure 10–5.

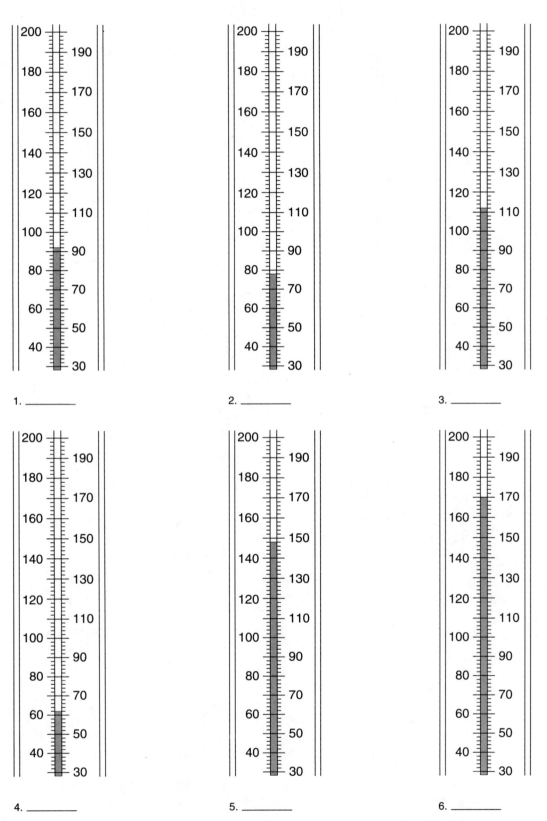

1. _____

2. _____

3. _____

4. _____

5. _____

6. _____

Figure 10–5

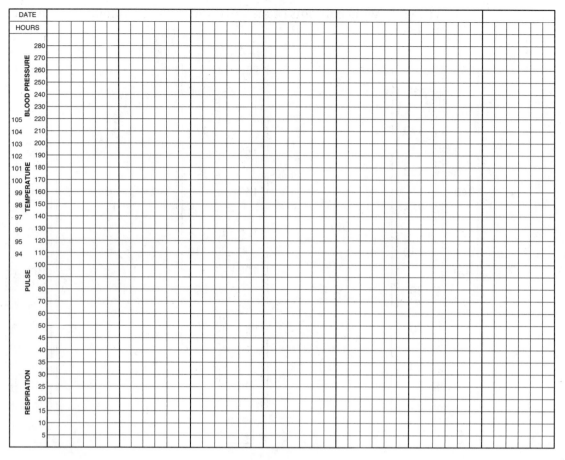

Figure 10–6

4. Graph the following vital signs on the graphic chart, Figure 10–6. Be sure to note the following information:

- How the temperature was taken if it was not oral—if the pulse was an apical pulse
- If the pulse or respirations were irregular
- Each set of vitals were taken at 0800 each day

Date	TPR	BP
12-16-XX	98.3 - 75 AP - 18	164/74
12-17-XX	99.4 - 83 irr - 16	170/86
12-18-XX	100.0 R - 88 - 18	158/66
12-19-XX	97.8 - 74 - 20	150/80

Role Play

Choose a nurse, a nursing assistant, and a patient for this role play. In the first part the nurse orders the nursing assistant to take vital signs on a patient. In the second part the nursing assistant goes to the patient and takes vital signs. In the third part the nursing assistant returns to the nurse and reports the vital signs for the patient. (Take care to use proper reporting form and to report reasonable vital signs. The vital signs should either be within the normal range or the abnormal vital signs should be noted. See the Language at Work at the end of this chapter for an example.)

THE PATIENT WITH OXYGEN

Vocabulary Sentences

1. I noticed that **Mrs. Ortega** has some irritation on her right nostril.
2. The oxygen **flowmeter** is set by the nurse.

CONDITIONS AND DISEASES

Vocabulary Sentences

1. If **strep throat** is left untreated, rheumatic fever may result.
2. A **chronic obstructive pulmonary disease** blocks the exchange of gases.
3. A patient with bronchitis often has a **productive cough**.
4. Mr. Black has **pneumonia**.
5. **Asthma** may cause a patient to have **wheezing** during expiration.
6. **Coronary artery disease** is a type of heart disease.
7. A **thrombus** can completely block the flow of blood to a body part.
8. **Angina** pain caused Mrs. Lopez to stop her activity and rest.
9. An **electrocardiogram** or **EKG** is done to help the doctor diagnose a **myocardial infarction**.
10. If a patient has a **cardiac arrest** the nursing assistant should call a code.
11. A patient with **pulmonary edema** must be observed for dyspnea and coughing up bloody sputum.
12. A patient who has hypertension may have a **cerebrovascular accident**.

Listening

Listen and circle the word you hear.

1. AX	AP	BP
2. accurate	oral	axillary
3. dilate	diastolic	systolic
4. bets	lets	sweats
5. sign	sing	sin
6. brain	vein	train
7. trachea	brachial	bronchi
8. freezing	wheezing	trees
9. hypertension	hypotension	hyperactive
10. inspiration	expiration	irritation
11. aorta	artery	alveoli

Medical Terminology

cardio-	heart
vascular-	blood vessels
circum-	circle, around
tachy-	fast
brady-	slow
hyper-	higher than normal
hypo-	lower than normal
-tension	blood pressure
cerebro-	brain

Combine the medical word parts above to make a word to fit each of the meanings below.

1. the body system that involves the heart and blood vessels

2. lower than normal blood pressure

_____

3. higher than normal blood pressure

_____

4. fast heart rate

_____

5. slow heart rate

_____

6. brain and blood vessels

_____

Find 4 other words in this chapter with "cardio" as a root and write the meaning of each.

1. _____

2. _____

3. _____

4. _____

The root "circum" is found in the words "circulate" and "circulatory system." How does the meaning of "circum" relate to the meanings of these 2 words?

_____

_____

_____

_____

_____

_____

_____

_____

_____

_____

LANGUAGE AT WORK

Part I

The nurse, Julia, asks the nursing assistant, Jose, to take vital signs on Mr. Callahan. He is a patient with COPD and has oxygen at 2 liters by nasal cannula.

Julia: Jose, Mr. Callahan needs his vital signs taken at 1600. You need to use the large size blood pressure cuff on him. The ear thermometer would be best because he's on O_2.

Jose: Do you want me to report his vital signs to you stat?

Julia: No, not unless there is anything unusual. His BP is usually about 165/90. Let me know if it's any higher than that.

Part II

Jose and Mr. Callahan

Jose: Mr. Callahan, I'm Jose, the nursing assistant. I'll be taking care of you. Can I check your identification bracelet?

Mr. Callahan: Hello. Yes, I'm Mr. Callahan.

Jose: How are you today?

Mr. Callahan: Not too bad. The oxygen is helping me breathe better.

Jose: Well, I'd like to take your vital signs. Is that OK with you?

Mr. Callahan: Certainly.

Part III

Jose took Mr. Callahan's vital signs and reports to Julia.

Jose: Julia, I would like to tell you about Mr. Callahan. First of all, he stated that his breathing is better now that he's on oxygen. He has no signs of cyanosis, but I thought that I should tell you about his vital signs. His TPR was 99.2, 96, 20. His BP was 180/100. Also, his pulse was irregular.

Julia: His pulse is usually irregular. His BP is awfully high. Why don't you chart those numbers while I go in and check on him.

Questions

1. What size blood pressure cuff is needed for Mr. Callahan?

   _____

2. How should his temperature be taken? Why is this method best?

   _____

3. Was Mr. Callahan's blood pressure higher than usual for him?

   _____

4. What was abnormal about his pulse?

   _____

COMPETENCY CHECKLIST 8: BEGINNING PROCEDURE ACTIONS

ACTIONS	SATISFACTORY	UNSATISFACTORY (COMMENTS)
Wash your hands.		
Bring equipment to room and knock on door.		
Ask visitors to leave and tell them where to wait.		
Identify patient, introduce yourself, explain and ask for cooperation.		
Close privacy curtains.		
Put on gloves if necessary.		
Raise bed to comfortable height, use good body mechanics.		

INSTRUCTOR'S SIGNATURE _____ DATE _____

COMPETENCY CHECKLIST 9: ENDING PROCEDURE ACTIONS

ACTIONS	SATISFACTORY	UNSATISFACTORY (COMMENTS)
Dispose of contaminated equipment. Remove gloves and wash hands.		
Lower bed to lowest position. Raise side rails.		
Make patient comfortable and give call button.		
Tell visitors they may enter.		
Write notes about what you did and your observations		
Report and document.		

INSTRUCTOR'S SIGNATURE _____ DATE _____

COMPETENCY CHECKLIST 10: TAKING THE TEMPERATURE

ACTIONS	SATISFACTORY	UNSATISFACTORY (COMMENTS)
Perform beginning procedure actions. Prepare thermometer.		
Place thermometer under tongue in patient's mouth.		
Remove glass thermometer after 3 minutes. Remove sheath or clean thermometer, hold at eye level and read.		
Remove electronic thermometer at the "beep." Dispose of probe cover and read display.		
For axillary temperature, place thermometer in center of armpit against skin.		
For rectal temperature prepare red probe or rectal glass thermometer and apply lubricant. Put on gloves.		
Position patient on side, insert thermometer 1½ inches into rectum and hold in place.		
Perform ending procedure actions.		

INSTRUCTOR'S SIGNATURE _____ DATE _____

COMPETENCY CHECKLIST 11: TAKING THE PULSE

ACTIONS	SATISFACTORY	UNSATISFACTORY (COMMENTS)
Perform beginning procedure actions. Place second and third fingers on radial artery (thumb side of inside of wrist).		
Count pulse for 1 minute. Note if irregular. Perform ending procedure actions.		

INSTRUCTOR'S SIGNATURE _____ DATE _____

COMPETENCY CHECKLIST 12: TAKING THE RESPIRATIONS

ACTIONS	SATISFACTORY	UNSATISFACTORY (COMMENTS)
Perform beginning procedure actions. Keep fingers in position on the pulse and look at chest rise and fall. Count for one minute. Note if irregular.		
If necessary, place patient's hand on his chest to help see chest rise and fall. Perform ending procedure actions.		

INSTRUCTOR'S SIGNATURE _____ DATE _____

COMPETENCY CHECKLIST 13: TAKING THE BLOOD PRESSURE

ACTIONS	SATISFACTORY	UNSATISFACTORY (COMMENTS)
Perform beginning procedure actions. Apply correct size cuff over brachial artery and feel for the brachial pulse.		
Then position fingers on radial pulse and inflate cuff until pulse is no longer felt. Note number and deflate cuff.		
Wait 15 seconds, position stethoscope over brachial artery and inflate cuff 30 mm of mercury above pressure noted above.		
Open screw slowly and listen for first strong beat. Continue to deflate cuff slowly until last strong beat is heard. Completely deflate cuff. Perform ending procedure actions.		

INSTRUCTOR'S SIGNATURE _____ DATE _____

Chapter 11: Skeletal System and the Muscular System/Moving and Positioning Patients

VOCABULARY

amputation
approximately
arthritis
atrophy
bedridden
cane
cast
centimeter
combative
compound fracture
constrict
contracture
crutches
cyanosis
daily
dangle
dependent patient
dilate
elevating
feet
foot board
fraction

fracture
gait
gangrene
geriatric chair
hand roll
height
inch
joint
kilogram
ligament
logroll
muscular system
nonambulatory
numbness
orthopedic injury
orthopedist
osteoarthritis
osteoporosis
paralyzed
paraplegic
passive

position the patient
postural support
pound
prosthesis
quadriplegic
range of motion
recliner
reduce the fracture
rheumatoid arthritis
scale
skeletal system
spinal cord
sprain
strain
swelling
tendon
traction
transfer
transport
walker
weight

ABBREVIATIONS

AKA	above the knee amputation	**ht**	height
amb	ambulatory	**in**	inches
BKA	below the knee amputation	**kg**	kilogram
cm	centimeter	**lb**	pound
ft	feet	**ROM**	range of motion
fx	fracture	**wt**	weight
geri chair	geriatric chair		

HOW THE SKELETAL SYSTEM AND THE MUSCULAR SYSTEM WORK TOGETHER

Vocabulary Sentences

1. The **skeletal system** and the **muscular system** work together to allow the body to move in many different ways.
2. The spine protects the **spinal cord**.
3. We exercise our **joints** through their normal **range of motion** during our daily activities.
4. When a patient is **bedridden** his muscles may **atrophy**.
5. **Foot boards** and **hand rolls** are used to prevent **contractures**.

Label the Diagram

Label the parts of the skeletal system on the diagram, Figure 11–1.

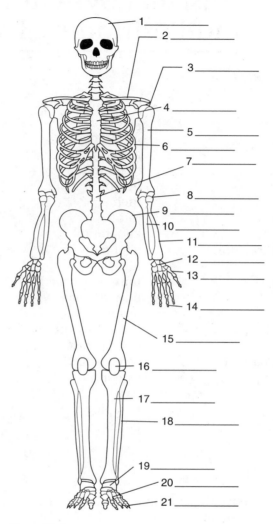

1 _____
2 _____
3 _____
4 _____
5 _____
6 _____
7 _____
8 _____
9 _____
10 _____
11 _____
12 _____
13 _____
14 _____
15 _____
16 _____
17 _____
18 _____
19 _____
20 _____
21 _____

Figure 11–1

Label the parts of the muscular system on the diagram, Figure 11–2.

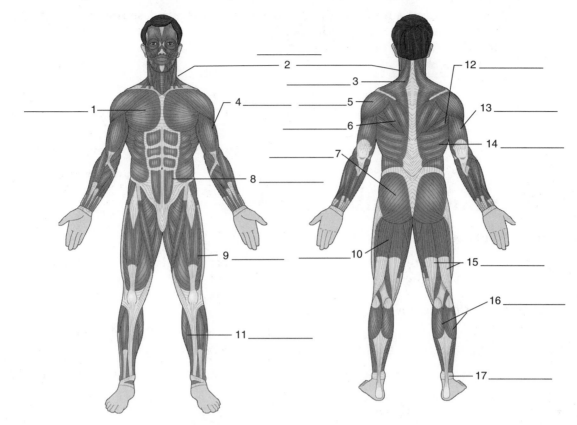

Figure 11–2

POSITIONING, TRANSFERRING, AMBULATING AND TRANSPORTING PATIENTS

Vocabulary Sentences

1. Many patients in hospitals and nursing homes are **dependent patients**.
2. One nursing assistant duty is to **position the patient**.
3. Sometimes it is necessary to **logroll** a patient because of his neck or back problem.
4. The nurse said, "Please **transfer** Mr. Packard from the bed to the chair."
5. An **ambulatory** patient may suddenly become **nonambulatory** while walking.
6. You can **transport** a patient by wheelchair or stretcher.

Discussion Questions

1. What should you do if you are helping a patient ambulate and he suddenly becomes nonambulatory?

Writing

Write 5 orders a nurse might give a nursing assistant. Use the following words at least once in the 5 orders: position, transport, transfer, ambulate. Example: Elif, please transfer Mrs. Vinton from the bed to the chair.

1. _____

2. _____

3. _____

4. _____

5. _____

MEASURING WEIGHT AND HEIGHT

Vocabulary Sentences

1. The nursing assistant measured Mr. Garcia's **height** in **centimenters**.
2. What is the patient's **weight** in **pounds**?

Fraction Review

Weight and height are measured in whole numbers and in parts of whole numbers called fractions. Let us use a circle to understand fractions, Figure 11–3.

If we have a circle and we cut it into two pieces we have two halves.

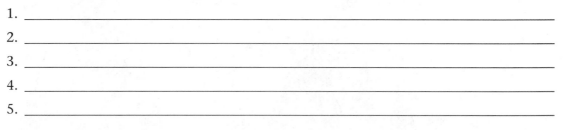

If we cut the circle in four we would have four quarters. (One of the American coins is called a quarter. How many quarters make a dollar?)

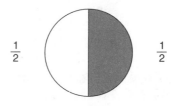

If we have two quarters, we call it one half.

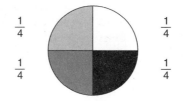

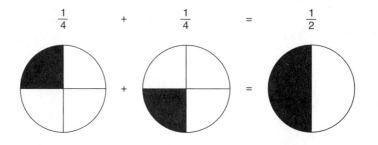

Figure 11–3

If we have three quarters, we call it three fourths.

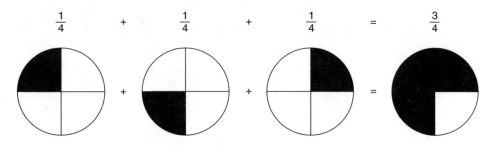

One half plus one quarter equals three fourths.

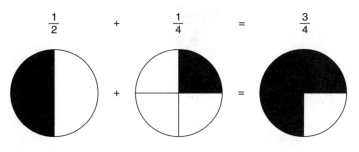

Figure 11–3 Continued.

Now try these fraction problems:

1. $\dfrac{1}{4} + \dfrac{1}{4} =$ _____

2. $\dfrac{1}{2} + \dfrac{1}{4} =$ _____

3. $\dfrac{1}{2} + \dfrac{1}{2} =$ _____

4. $\dfrac{1}{4} + \dfrac{1}{4} + \dfrac{1}{4} =$ _____

Short Answer

1. Write the weight shown on the following scales on the line beside each scale, Figure 11–4.

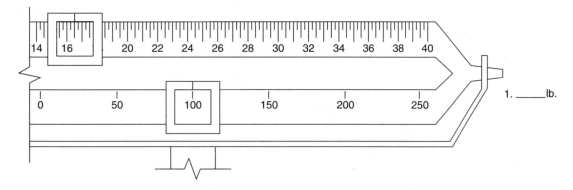

Figure 11–4

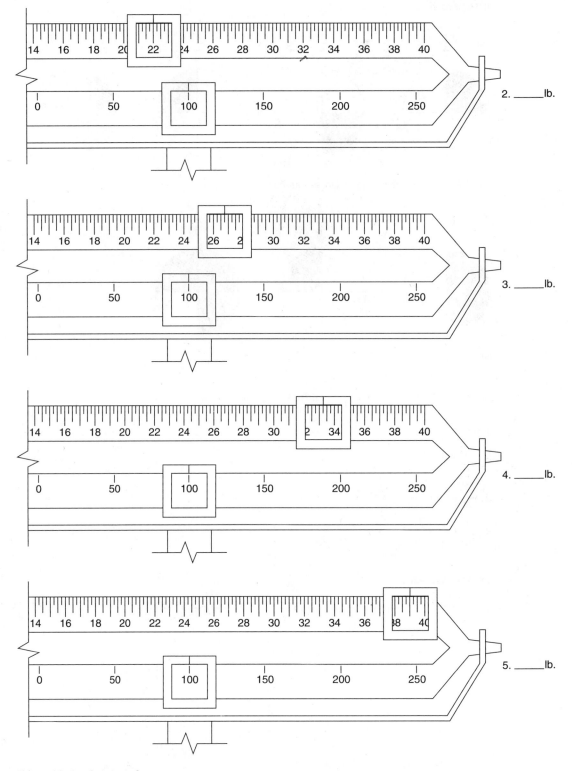

2. _____ lb.

3. _____ lb.

4. _____ lb.

5. _____ lb.

Figure 11–4 Continued.

2. Write the height in inches and also in feet and inches shown on the following scales, Figure 11–5.

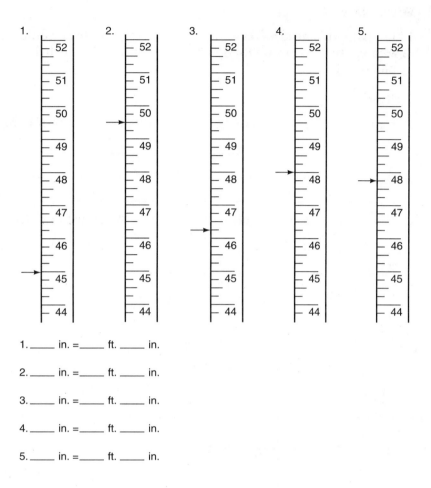

1. ____ in. = ____ ft. ____ in.

2. ____ in. = ____ ft. ____ in.

3. ____ in. = ____ ft. ____ in.

4. ____ in. = ____ ft. ____ in.

5. ____ in. = ____ ft. ____ in.

Figure 11–5

Circle Dialogues

Circle dialogues are to be done as a class. Try to remember the line without looking at the book. To have fun with the exercise, make up a funny height and weight for yourself. Continue around the class until everyone has had a turn.

Part 1: Height
Student A: How tall are you?
Student B: I am _____.
(Turns to the next student and reads the line for student A.)

Part 2: Weight

Student A: How much do you weigh?
Student B: I weigh _____. (Turns to next person.)
              What is your weight?
Student C: My weight is _____.
(Turns to next person and reads the line for student A.)

RESTRAINTS AND POSTURAL SUPPORTS

Vocabulary Sentences

1. If a patient is **combative** there is the danger that he could hurt himself or others.
2. A **postural support** or **geriatric chair** may be helpful for a patient who is paralyzed.

Writing

1. Name 3 different types of restraints and tell why each one might be used.

    1. _____

    2. _____

    3. _____

2. What are 4 safety measures you must take when using restraints on a patient?

    1. _____

    2. _____

    3. _____

    4. _____

3. What can long-term care facilities do to reduce the use of restraints on residents?

    _____

    _____

    _____

CONDITIONS AND DISEASES

Vocabulary Sentences

1. A **fracture** can be very painful.
2. The **orthopedist** decides how to **reduce the fracture** so that the bones will heal properly.
3. **Sprains** and **strains** are common sport injuries.
4. Injuries to **ligaments** and **tendons** do not show on X-rays.
5. **Osteoarthritis** and **rheumatoid arthritis** are 2 kinds of **arthritis**.
6. Patients with **osteoporosis** may become shorter and more hunched over.
7. **Amputation** is often necessary when a patient has **gangrene**.

Listening

Listen and circle the word you hear in each line.

1. orthopedist   orthodontist   osteoporosis
2. sprain   strain   stain
3. fracture   factual   fraction
4. skeletal   skeleton   skull
5. height   weight   gait

TREATMENT OF ORTHOPEDIC PROBLEMS

Vocabulary Sentences

1. Applying cold packs makes blood vessels **constrict**.
2. Heat makes blood vessels **dilate**.

3. A fractured arm or leg is often put in a **cast**.
4. **Cyanosis** and **numbness** occur when there is not enough blood circulation.
5. **Traction** is usually necessary for a fractured femur.
6. Patients with spinal cord injuries may be **paraplegic** or **quadriplegic**.

Medical Terminology

arthr-   joint
-itis   inflammation
myo-   muscle
osteo-   bone
-plegia paralysis (not being able to move)
quadri- 4

Separate the following words into word parts and write the meaning of each part and the whole word.

1. arthritis

_____

2. osteoarthritis

_____

3. quadriplegia

_____

LANGUAGE AT WORK

A nurse asks a nursing assistant to weigh and measure a patient.

RN: Please take Mr. Smith's weight and height and then have him wait in exam room 3 for the doctor.
NA: OK, I'll weigh and measure him and have him wait in room 3.
NA: Mr. Smith?
Pt.:   Yes?
NA: Mr. Smith, may I check your ID band? I need to take your weight and height. Would you come this way, please? Please step up on the scale.
Pt.:   How much do I weigh?
NA: You weigh 155 pounds.
Pt.:   How tall am I?
NA: You are five feet nine and one half inches.
Pt.:   Do you think I weigh too much?
NA: Well, you'll have to talk to Dr. Simms about that. If you'll wait here in room 3, the doctor will be in to see you shortly.

Questions

1. How tall is Mr. Smith?

_____

2. Was the nursing assistant right not to discuss Mr. Smith's weight with him? Why?

_____

3. What does "see you shortly" mean?

_____

COMPETENCY CHECKLIST 14: PASSIVE RANGE OF MOTION EXERCISES

ACTIONS	SATISFACTORY	UNSATISFACTORY (COMMENTS)
Perform beginning procedure actions. Move the shoulder.		
Move the elbow.		
Move the wrist.		
Move the fingers.		
Move the hip and knee.		
Move the foot and toes. Perform ending procedure actions.		

INSTRUCTOR'S SIGNATURE _____ DATE _____

COMPETENCY CHECKLIST 15: MOVING A PATIENT UP IN BED

ACTIONS	SATISFACTORY	UNSATISFACTORY (COMMENTS)
Perform beginning procedure actions. Place pillow at head of bed. Place turning sheet under shoulders and hips.		
Roll sheet close to body. Patient should bend knees and cross arms on chest.		
NAs use good body mechanics on count of 3 to lift and move patient to head of bed.		
Place pillow under head, straighten turning sheet and make patient comfortable.		
One NA may move small patient by using arm and leg muscles to lift. Perform ending procedure actions.		

INSTRUCTOR'S SIGNATURE _____ DATE _____

COMPETENCY CHECKLIST 16:
TURNING A PATIENT IN BED ONTO HIS SIDE

ACTIONS	SATISFACTORY	UNSATISFACTORY (COMMENTS)
Perform beginning procedure actions. Cross patient's far leg over near leg and far arm over chest. Turn patient toward you.		
Raise side rail, go to other side and lower side rail. Place your hands first under upper body and then under lower body and pull patient to center of bed.		
Place pillows at back, under upper arm and between legs and ankles.		
2 NAs can use turning sheet to move patient to left side of bed. Then turn patient onto right side and place pillows as above. Perform ending procedure actions.		

INSTRUCTOR'S SIGNATURE _____ DATE _____

COMPETENCY CHECKLIST 17: LOG-ROLLING A PATIENT IN BED

ACTIONS	SATISFACTORY	UNSATISFACTORY (COMMENTS)
Perform beginning procedure actions. Place pillow between legs. Two NAs are on left side and 1 NA is on right side of bed. Move patient toward left side with turning sheet.		
One NA goes to right side of bed.		
Two NAs roll patient toward them. Position pillows for comfort. Perform ending procedure actions.		

INSTRUCTOR'S SIGNATURE _____ DATE _____

COMPETENCY CHECKLIST 18: TRANSFERRING A PATIENT FROM BED TO CHAIR OR TO WHEELCHAIR

ACTIONS	SATISFACTORY	UNSATISFACTORY (COMMENTS)
Perform beginning procedure actions. Raise head of bed to sit patient up. Place wheelchair near stronger side. Lock wheels, raise footrests. Allow patient to dangle.		
Apply transfer belt. NA holds belt and patient holds onto NA's shoulders. Lift, turn, and assist patient into chair. Perform ending procedure actions.		

INSTRUCTOR'S SIGNATURE _____ DATE _____

COMPETENCY CHECKLIST 19: TRANSFERRING A PATIENT FROM STRETCHER TO BED OR WHEELCHAIR

ACTIONS	SATISFACTORY	UNSATISFACTORY (COMMENTS)
Perform beginning procedure actions. Place stretcher and bed at same height and lock wheels. Four NAs roll bottom sheet of stretcher close to patient's body.		
On count of 3 lift and move patient onto bed.		
Roll patient onto left side. Push sheets under the body.		
Roll patient onto right side. Pull out sheets.		
Cover patient and make comfortable.		
If slider is available, place slider under sheets of stretcher.		

COMPETENCY CHECKLIST 19: TRANSFERRING A PATIENT FROM STRETCHER TO BED (CONTINUED)

ACTIONS	SATISFACTORY	UNSATISFACTORY (COMMENTS)
Grasp slider and pull patient onto bed. Roll patient onto side to remove slider. Perform ending procedure actions.		

INSTRUCTOR'S SIGNATURE _____ DATE _____

COMPETENCY CHECKLIST 20: USING A MECHANICAL LIFT

ACTIONS	SATISFACTORY	UNSATISFACTORY (COMMENTS)
Perform beginning procedure actions. Note the lift and the sling.		
To position sling, 2 NAs roll patient onto left side and place folded sling against body.		
Roll patient onto right side and straighten sling.		
Sling reaches from shoulders to knees.		
Position lift over bed. Attach hooks with open ends away from body.		
Raise lift and swing patient to chair. One NA can support legs.		
Lower lift and seat patient in chair. Make comfortable. Perform ending procedure actions.		

INSTRUCTOR'S SIGNATURE _____ DATE _____

COMPETENCY CHECKLIST 21:
EASING A FALLING PATIENT TO THE FLOOR

ACTIONS	SATISFACTORY	UNSATISFACTORY (COMMENTS)
Grasp patient under arms and hold onto arms at the wrist. Place your leg and upper body against patient's back.		
If patient is wearing gait belt, hold onto it. Place your leg and upper body against patient's back.		
Ease patient to floor. Support head, stay with patient, call for help. Do not move patient until nurse tells you to do so.		

INSTRUCTOR'S SIGNATURE _____ DATE _____

COMPETENCY CHECKLIST 22: TRANSPORTING A PATIENT
BY WHEELCHAIR OR BY STRETCHER

ACTIONS	SATISFACTORY	UNSATISFACTORY (COMMENTS)
Perform beginning procedure actions. Push from head of stretcher. Stay to right in hallways.		
Stand behind wheelchair and push it forward.		
Going down a ramp, stand at foot of stretcher to control it.		
Going down a ramp, back wheelchair down.		
When using elevator, push "stop" button when entering and exiting. Push "start" button after leaving elevator.		
When entering elevator with stretcher, back it in. To exit, push it out.		
When entering elevator with wheelchair, back it in.		

COMPETENCY CHECKLIST 22: TRANSPORTING A PATIENT BY WHEELCHAIR OR BY STRETCHER (CONTINUED)

ACTIONS	SATISFACTORY	UNSATISFACTORY (COMMENTS)
When exiting elevator, back wheelchair out.		
Lock wheels of wheelchair or stretcher when arriving at new place.		
Give report about the patient to another health care worker. Perform ending procedure actions.		

INSTRUCTOR'S SIGNATURE _____ DATE _____

COMPETENCY CHECKLIST 23: MEASURING A PATIENT'S WEIGHT

ACTIONS	SATISFACTORY	UNSATISFACTORY (COMMENTS)
Perform beginning procedure actions. Raise height bar and ask patient to step onto scale.		
Slide small and large weight indicator to "0."		
Slide large weight indicator to right. Do not allow balance bar to touch bottom.		
Move small weight indicator slowly to right until balance bar hangs in the middle. Perform ending procedure actions.		

INSTRUCTOR'S SIGNATURE _____ DATE _____

COMPETENCY CHECKLIST 24: MEASURING A PATIENT'S HEIGHT

ACTIONS	SATISFACTORY	UNSATISFACTORY (COMMENTS)
Perform beginning procedure actions. Assist patient to stand on scale with back toward height bar.		
Lower height bar to top of head.		
Read the height bar at top of head. If taller than 51 inches, read bar at break in the bar. Assist patient off scale. Perform ending procedure actions.		

INSTRUCTOR'S SIGNATURE _____ DATE _____

COMPETENCY CHECKLIST 25: USING RESTRAINTS

ACTIONS	SATISFACTORY	UNSATISFACTORY (COMMENTS)
Perform beginning procedure actions. Explain procedure calmly to patient.		
Secure ties to frame of mattress where patient cannot reach them.		
Tie a knot that can be released quickly. Perform ending procedure actions.		

INSTRUCTOR'S SIGNATURE _____ DATE _____

Chapter 12: Integumentary System/Caring for the Patient's Personal Needs

VOCABULARY

admitted
barber
beard
blister
buttocks
classified
commode
dentures
dermis
discharged
eczema
epidermis
fracture bedpan
gland
groom
hair follicle
herpes simplex

hydrated
impetigo
incontinent
lotion
lubricated
making a bed
melanin
nail bed
nourished
occupied
ointment
palm
partial
perineum
pore
pressure ulcer

progress
promptly
receptacle
request
scar
sebum
sensation
shampoo
shearing
skin breakdown
sole
supply
tangle
waterproof
whirlpool
wrinkle

ABBREVIATIONS

DC'd   discharged
NPO   nothing by mouth
peri care   care of the perineum
postop   after the operation
PRN   as necessary

FUNCTIONS AND PARTS OF THE INTEGUMENTARY SYSTEM

Vocabulary Sentences

1. The **epidermis** contains **melanin**, which gives the skin its color.
2. The thickness of the **dermis** changes in different parts of the body.
3. All of the skin on our bodies contains **hair follicles** except for the **palms** of our hands and the **soles** of our feet.
4. The oil **gland** in the skin produces **sebum**.
5. Perspiration is released through the **pores** in our skin.
6. The **nail bed** grows nails to protect the ends of our fingers and toes.

Label the Diagram

Label the parts of the integumentary system on the diagram, Figure 12–1.

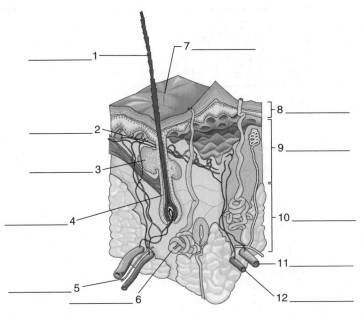

Figure 12–1

CARE OF THE INTEGUMENTARY SYSTEM

Vocabulary Sentences

1. Good skin care prevents **skin breakdown**.
2. **Partial** bedbaths are given daily and whenever necessary.
3. **Incontinent** patients must be given frequent skin care.
4. Keeping well **hydrated** and **nourished** helps prevent **pressure ulcers**.
5. When giving a bedbath be sure to change the water before and after **peri care.**
6. A nursing assistant may be expected to **groom** a patient's hair.

Culture Exchange

Answer the following questions by yourself or with someone from your birth country. Then compare answers with your classmates.

1. In your country, who takes care of a patient's personal needs when they are unable to take care of themselves?

   _____

2. Have you ever taken care of the personal needs of someone? Who? How did you feel about it?

   _____

3. How do you feel about taking care of the personal needs of a stranger? How would you feel about having a stranger take care of your personal needs?

   _____

   _____

4. As a nursing assistant, what can you do to help a patient feel more comfortable about having a stranger take care of her personal needs?

   _____

   _____

TAKING CARE OF THE OTHER PERSONAL HYGIENE NEEDS OF THE PATIENT

Vocabulary Sentences

1. Mouth care includes keeping the lips **lubricated.**
2. **Dentures** need special care and careful handling.
3. The **fracture bedpan** can be slipped under a patient's **buttocks**.
4. The **commode** has a removable **receptacle** that must be disinfected after use.

What Do You Say?

Write an appropriate response for a nursing assistant to make to each of the following sentences.

1. Can you help me here? I really need to pee.

   _____

2. I can wash my own private parts.

   _____

3. I have a sore area on my bottom.

   _____

4. My hands are feeling so dry.

   _____

5. They won't let me get up yet, but I really feel the need to use the facilities.

   _____

MAKING THE PATIENT'S BED

Vocabulary Sentences

1. A closed bed is made when a patient has been **discharged.**
2. An open bed is made when a patient is to be **admitted.**
3. An **occupied bed** is made when a patient is bedridden.
4. A **postop** bed is made when a patient will be returning from surgery.

Listening

Listen to each sentence. Then circle the phrase you heard.

1. a. make an occupied bed
   b. make an unoccupied bed
   c. make a postop bed
2. a. transfer Mr. Joel
   b. transfer Mr. Jones
   c. transfer Mrs. Joel
3. a. in room 106
   b. in room 116
   c. in room 160
4. a. bedbath, shampoo, and mouth care
   b. shampoo, shower, and mouth care
   c. bedbath, shower, and mouth care
5. a. lower left buttock
   b. lower left quadrant
   c. lower left back

CONDITIONS AND DISEASES

Vocabulary Sentences

1. A red area can **progress** to an open area in the skin.
2. Burns are **classified** by how deeply they affect the skin.
3. **Eczema** is treated with **ointments**.
4. Cold sores are caused by the **herpes simplex** virus.
5. **Impetigo** is very contagious.

Role Play

Choose 2 nursing assistants for this role play. The first nursing assistant has more work than she has time to finish. The second nursing assistant is done with his work and is reading procedure manuals. The first nursing assistant asks the second nursing assistant for help finishing her work. The work should include at least 2 procedures from this chapter. Start from the following line or use your own.

Peggy: Hi Tim. Are you learning interesting things from the procedure manual?

Medical Terminology

1. Separate the word "epidermis" into a prefix and root. Write the meaning of each.

   Prefix _____   Meaning _____

   Root _____   Meaning _____

LANGUAGE AT WORK

Two nursing assistants discuss how much work they have and learn to ask for help.

Kim: Lee, I have 4 total care patients today. Do you think that you could help me with Mrs. Greenberg in room 610?

Lee: Sure Kim, I'd be glad to help you out. I have a light assignment today, not a heavy one like yours.

Kim: Mrs. Greenberg is incontinent and has the beginning of a pressure ulcer on her right buttock. I'll tell the nurse about that red area when I give her report. Can you get me a basin of water, washcloth and towel, and some clean linen so I can clean her before turning her onto her left side?

Lee: No problem, Kim. I wish that you had asked me to help you out sooner. One of my patients was self care and one was partial care. So, I have nothing left to do until the lunch trays arrive.

Questions

1. How many total care patients does Kim have today?

   _____

2. Does Lee have total care or self care patients today?

   _____

3. Does Kim have a light assignment or a heavy assignment today?

   _____

Continued on next page.

4. On what part of the body is Mrs. Greenberg's pressure ulcer?

_____

5. Onto what side should Kim and Lee turn Mrs. Greenberg now?

_____

6. What can Lee do to help Kim out? Why does Lee have extra time today?

_____

COMPETENCY CHECKLIST 26: GIVING A BEDBATH

ACTIONS	SATISFACTORY	UNSATISFACTORY (COMMENTS)
Perform beginning procedure actions. Remove gown and cover patient with bath blanket.		
Make a mitt with washcloth.		
Wash face. Start with eyes. Do not use soap. Wash ears and neck.		
Place towel under arms and wash. Apply deodorant.		
Wash chest and under breasts of woman.		
Leave towel on chest, lower bath blanket and wash abdomen.		
Place towel under legs and wash.		
Place foot in basin or wash with washcloth. Wash and dry between toes. Apply lotion to heels.		
For male: Change water and washcloth. Raise bath blanket up to waist and bring up top linens to cover legs and expose genitals. Wear gloves and wash from tip of penis to scrotum.		
Push back foreskin if necessary.		

COMPETENCY CHECKLIST 26: GIVING A BEDBATH (CONTINUED)

ACTIONS	SATISFACTORY	UNSATISFACTORY (COMMENTS)
For female: Change water and washcloth. Wear gloves. Arrange bath blanket with corners pointing to head and feet and side corners wrapped around legs. Lift bottom corner to expose genitals.		
Spread vulva and wash with downward strokes.		
Turn patient on side. Wash rectal area, wiping up toward rectum.		
Change water and gloves. Lay towel along back and wash back, neck and upper part of legs.		
Place lotion on hands and rub together. Give gentle backrub.		
Dry back with towel Pat powder onto back. Turn patient onto back, give hair care, mouth care, make the bed. Perform ending procedure actions.		

INSTRUCTOR'S SIGNATURE _____ DATE _____

COMPETENCY CHECKLIST 27: SHAVING A MALE PATIENT

ACTIONS	SATISFACTORY	UNSATISFACTORY (COMMENTS)
Perform beginning procedure actions. Prepare basin with warm water and wash cloth. Wear gloves. Wet face and apply shaving cream.		
Hold skin with one hand. Use short strokes with razor in direction of hair growth. Start on side of face, near ear. Rinse razor frequently. Perform ending procedure actions.		

INSTRUCTOR'S SIGNATURE _____ DATE _____

COMPETENCY CHECKLIST 28: GIVING FINGERNAIL CARE

ACTIONS	SATISFACTORY	UNSATISFACTORY (COMMENTS)
Perform beginning procedure actions. Soak fingernails in basin of warm water for 10 or 15 minutes.		
Clip nails. Use emery board to round corners.		
Use orangewood stick to clean under nails and push down cuticles. Apply lotion. Perform ending procedure actions.		

INSTRUCTOR'S SIGNATURE _____ DATE _____

COMPETENCY CHECKLIST 29: GIVING FOOT AND TOENAIL CARE

ACTIONS	SATISFACTORY	UNSATISFACTORY (COMMENTS)
Perform beginning procedure actions. Soak each foot in basin of warm water for 10 to 15 minutes.		
Dry feet well. Look for red or open areas. Use orangewood stick to clean under nails.		
Apply lotion to heels. Perform ending procedure actions.		

INSTRUCTOR'S SIGNATURE _____ DATE _____

COMPETENCY CHECKLIST 30: GIVING ORAL HYGIENE

ACTIONS	SATISFACTORY	UNSATISFACTORY (COMMENTS)
Perform beginning procedure actions. Sit patient up and place towel around neck. Wear gloves, apply toothpaste to a wet toothbrush.		
Assist patient to brush teeth.		
Floss teeth with floss wrapped around middle fingers.		
Patient can rinse mouth and spit into emesis basin. Mouthwash can be used to rinse mouth.		
Lips may be lubricated with petroleum jelly.		
Assist patient in removing dentures using gauze and gloves.		
Place paper towel in sink and fill partially with cool or warm water. Brush dentures. Put dentures in denture cup with water.		
For unconscious patient, turn head to side. Use swabs and tongue depressor to clean mouth. Apply petroleum jelly to lips. Perform ending procedure actions.		

INSTRUCTOR'S SIGNATURE _____ DATE _____

COMPETENCY CHECKLIST 31: GIVING A PATIENT A BEDPAN

ACTIONS	SATISFACTORY	UNSATISFACTORY (COMMENTS)
Perform beginning procedure actions. Lower head of bed. Wear gloves, assist patient to raise hips, and place bedpan and chux under buttocks.		
Another method is to turn patient away from you. Place bedpan against buttocks and roll him onto bedpan.		
Raise head of bed and side rails. Give patient call button.		
Lower head of bed. Have patient raise hips to pull bedpan out. Or, turn him onto the side, holding onto bedpan.		
Roll toilet paper around gloved hands. Wipe perineum up toward rectum. Wash peri area if necessary.		
Raise side rails and carry covered bedpan into bathroom for disposal. Observe contents. Return cleaned bedpan to bedside table.		
After removing gloves and washing hands, record information on proper form. Perform ending procedure actions.		

INSTRUCTOR'S SIGNATURE _____ DATE _____

COMPETENCY CHECKLIST 32: UNDRESSING AND DRESSING A PATIENT

ACTIONS	SATISFACTORY	UNSATISFACTORY (COMMENTS)
Perform beginning procedure actions. If patient is dependent, put bed in flat position. Cover patient with clean gown. Remove dirty gown from strong side first, then weak side.		
Put clean gown on weak side, then strong side. Reach your arm through sleeve and pull out patient's arm.		
If patient is wearing pullover, roll patient onto weak side. Remove top from strong arm first.		
Turn patient onto other side. Remove pullover from weak arm.		
Slip pullover over head. Cover patient with sheet.		
To remove pants, have patient raise hips.		
If patient is dependent, turn him onto weak side and pull pants off hip of strong side first.		
Turn patient onto strong side and remove pants from hip of weak side.		
With patient on his back, both pants legs can be pulled down at same time.		
To put pants on, slide pants legs over patient's feet and lower legs. Roll patient from side to side to pull pants up. If patient is able, he can lift hips so you can pull pants up.		

COMPETENCY CHECKLIST 32:
UNDRESSING AND DRESSING A PATIENT (CONTINUED)

ACTIONS	SATISFACTORY	UNSATISFACTORY (COMMENTS)
To put pullover top on, pull it over head. Turn patient onto strong side. Gather up sleeve, put your arm through and grasp weak arm and pull it through. Turn patient onto other side and do same for strong arm.		
Socks are rolled up and placed over toes, then pulled up.		
Laces of shoes are opened completely to slip foot in. Tie securely. Perform ending procedure actions.		

INSTRUCTOR'S SIGNATURE _____ DATE _____

COMPETENCY CHECKLIST 33: MAKING A BED

ACTIONS	SATISFACTORY	UNSATISFACTORY (COMMENTS)
Perform beginning procedure actions. Remove dirty linens from bed. Wear gloves if they might be soiled with body fluids. Roll them together and put in laundry hamper. Unfold bottom sheet and place center fold at center of bed.		
Unfold bottom sheet. Place bottom edge of sheet at bottom edge of mattress.		
Make a corner.		
Place center fold of draw sheet at center of bed and unfold so that it will be under patient from shoulders to hips. Tuck it under mattress.		

COMPETENCY CHECKLIST 33: MAKING A BED (CONTINUED)

ACTIONS	SATISFACTORY	UNSATISFACTORY (COMMENTS)
Place center fold of top sheet in center of bed. Place top edge of sheet at top edge of mattress. Do same with blanket.		
Tuck under top sheet and blanket together at foot of bed and make a corner. Do not tuck under long edge, let it hang down.		
Go to other side of bed. Start with bottom sheet. Pull tight. Tuck it under top edge of mattress and make corner.		
Pull out draw sheet and tuck under mattress. Do same for top sheet and blanket. Make corner at foot of bed. Make cuff at head of bed by folding down top sheet and blanket.		
Fold pillow in half and push it into pillowcase. Do not put it against your uniform. Perform ending procedure actions.		

INSTRUCTOR'S SIGNATURE _____ DATE _____

COMPETENCY CHECKLIST 34: MAKING AN OCCUPIED BED

ACTIONS	SATISFACTORY	UNSATISFACTORY (COMMENTS)
Perform beginning procedure actions. Turn patient away from you onto side and push dirty linens underneath back.		
Make bed on one side.		
Raise side rail and turn patient toward you.		
Go to other side of bed, lower side rail, pull out dirty sheets and place in hamper. Pull out clean bottom sheet and draw sheet and make bed.		
Turn patient onto back. Lift head and shoulders to take out pillow. Change pillowcase and replace pillow under head.		
Place clean top sheet over dirty top sheet and blanket. Pull out dirty linen from underneath. Place blanket on top. Tuck blanket and top sheet under mattress and make corner. Fold cuff under patient' chin. Go to other side and complete bed. Perform ending procedure actions.		

INSTRUCTOR'S SIGNATURE _____ DATE _____

Chapter 13: Digestive System/Providing Nutrition to the Patient

VOCABULARY

absorption
anorexia nervosa
appendectomy
appendicitis
appendix
appetite
ascites
benign
bile
bowel
brief
broth
bulimia
calorie
cholecystitis
cholesterol
cleanse
colon
colonoscopy
colostomy
coma
constipated
culture and sensitivity
custard
defecation
dehydrated
detoxifying
diabetic diet
digestion
distended
duodenum
endoscopy
epiglottis
esophagus
estimate

fiber
flatus
food poisoning
force fluids
gallbladder
gastroenteritis
gastroscopy
gastrostomy
gavage
gelatin
ginger ale
guaiac
hematemesis
hepatic coma
ileostomy
ingestion
intake
intravenous
IV site
jaundice
label
large intestine
lavage
laxative
liver
malignant
melena
menu
metastasize
nasogastric
nausea
nourishments
nutrient
occult
output

ova and parasites
pancreas
peristalsis
peritoneum
peritonitis
popsicle
progresses
projection
protein
pudding
puree
restrict fluids
restricted
retention
rupture
saliva
semiformed
small intestine
sodium
source
specimen
stimulate
stoma
stomach
stool
strict
suction
suppository
therapeutic
tumor
ulcer
vacant
villus

ABBREVIATIONS

BM	bowel movement
cc	cubic centimeter
C&S	culture and sensitivity
I&O	intake and output
IV	intravenous
mL	milliliter
NAS	no added salt

NG	nasogastric
O&P	ova and parasites
oz	ounce
po	by mouth
preop	before the operation
SSE	soap suds enema
TPN	total parenteral nutrition

HOW THE DIGESTIVE SYSTEM FUNCTIONS

Vocabulary Sentences

1. The digestive system breaks down food into **nutrients** our cells can use.
2. The 4 main functions of the digestive system are **ingestion, digestion, absorption,** and **defecation.**
3. **Saliva** starts to digest food in the mouth.
4. The **esophagus** connects the mouth to the stomach.
5. The **epiglottis** prevents food from getting into the trachea.
6. **Peristalsis** pushes the food through the digestive system.
7. The **small intestine** is about 20 feet long.
8. **Bile** is stored in the **gallbladder.**
9. The **liver detoxifies** drugs and alcohol.
10. The **pancreas** is a gland that has many functions.
11. The wall of each **villus** is only 1 cell thick.
12. The **large intestine** is also called the **colon** and the **bowel.**
13. Did Mr. Ryan have a **bowel movement** today?
14. When an infection occurs in the **appendix** it is called **appendicitis.**

Label the Diagram

Label the parts of the digestive system on the diagram, Figure 13–1.

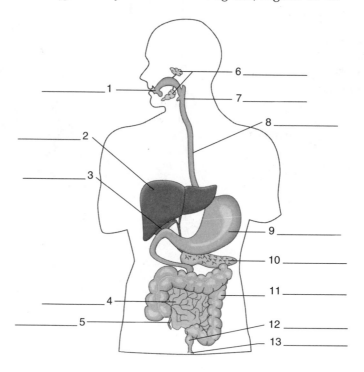

Figure 13–1

HELPING THE PATIENT MEET NUTRITIONAL NEEDS

Vocabulary Sentences

1. **Therapeutic** diets are ordered by the doctor.
2. Sometimes a patient's diet needs to be **restricted** in some way.
3. When a patient has **diarrhea** or is **preop**, he may be NPO.
4. **Dehydration** can be a life-threatening condition.
5. Clear liquids include **broth, ginger ale, gelatin**, and **popsicles.**
6. A full liquid diet may include **custard, pudding,** and **pureed** foods.
7. Patients with high blood pressure may be on a **sodium**-restricted diet.
8. A high **protein** diet may be used for a burn victim.
9. A **diabetic diet** restricts the amount of food and sugar.
10. Many people today try to eat less **cholesterol.**
11. Patients who are trying to lose weight may eat a low **calorie** diet.
12. Whole grain breads and dried fruit are high in **fiber.**
13. A patient's **appetite** is affected by how food is served.
14. **Gavage** feedings are given through the **nasogastric** tube.
15. Please observe Ms. Hall for **nausea** when you feed her.
16. A nasogastric tube can also be used to **suction** the stomach.
17. A **gastrostomy** may be necessary for a patient in a **coma.**

Matching

Match the therapeutic diet with the food a patient receives.

___1. clear liquid

___2. diabetic

___3. full liquid

___4. high residue

___5. light

___6. NPO

___7. sodium restricted

___8. soft

a. balanced diet that avoids simple sugars
b. contains only enough sodium for good nutrition
c. liquids that provide full nutrition
d. liquids that you can see through
e. foods with a great deal of fiber
f. mild in flavor, low in fiber and fat
g. not much fiber, easily digested and chewed
h. nothing by mouth, only intravenous nutrition

Short Answer

Intake Section of Intake and Output Form

Time	Oral		Tube Feeding	Intravenous	Other
	Kind	Amount			
8 Hour Total					
8 Hour Total					
8 Hour Total					
24 Hour Total					

Figure 13–2

Recording Intake. Record the following day of oral intake on the form provided in Figure 13–2.

The following cups, bowls, and glasses are used in the facility:

juice glass	150 cc
bowl	250 cc
coffee cup	200 cc
carton of milk	240 cc
custard, ice cream, and gelatin	125 cc

8:00 AM Breakfast	1 juice glass orange juice
	1 bowl of dry cereal with 1 small carton milk
	½ cup of coffee
	1 piece of toast
10:00 AM Snack	1 juice glass cranberry juice
12:00 noon Lunch	1 juice glass of ginger ale
	1 ham and cheese sandwich
	½ bowl of soup
	1 cup of ice cream
4:30 PM Snack	1 cup of coffee
	2 graham crackers
6:00 PM Dinner	1 chicken breast
	1 serving rice
	½ bowl gelatin
	½ juice glass apple juice

ELIMINATION FROM THE GASTROINTESTINAL SYSTEM

Vocabulary Sentences

1. A stool **specimen** may be taken for a **culture and sensitivity** test or an **ova and parasites** test.
2. A common name for a stool occult blood test is **guaiac** test.
3. The nurse may give the patient a **suppository** as part of a bowel retraining program.
4. An enema is used to **cleanse** the colon and rectum of stool and **flatus.**
5. If a patient is **constipated,** an enema may be ordered.
6. An oil-**retention** enema softens the stool.

Role Play

Choose a nursing assistant and a patient to act out the following scene. The nursing assistant has been assigned to bring dinner to a patient who has not eaten much all day. The nursing assistant goes in to see the patient before bringing the tray. Then the nursing assistant brings the tray in. The patient is tired and in pain and not really hungry. See Language at Work at the end of this chapter for words or phrases to use.

CONDITIONS AND DISEASES

Vocabulary Sentences

1. When food is the **source** of **gastroenteritis,** it is called **food poisoning.**
2. **Peritonitis** occurs when the appendix **ruptures** before an **appendectomy** is done.
3. A **distended** abdomen is one sign of an intestinal obstruction.
4. A **tumor** may be either **malignant** or **benign.**
5. I know Mr. Smith has a **stoma,** but is it a **colostomy** or an **ileostomy**?
6. If not diagnosed early, cancer can **mestatasize** to other organs.
7. **Gastroscopy** and **colonoscopy** are 2 types of **endoscopy.**
8. Gallstones are one cause of **cholecystitis.**
9. Most **ulcers** occur in the **duodenum** or stomach.
10. **Hematemesis** and **melena** are 2 symptoms of ulcers.
11. **Jaundice** and **ascites** develop in a person with cirrhosis, and a **hepatic coma** often causes death.
12. **Anorexia nervosa** and **bulimia** are 2 eating disorders.

Matching

Match the condition or disease with the symptoms or definition of the disease.

___1. anorexia

___2. appendicitis

___3. bulimia

___4. cholecystitis

___5. fecal impaction

___6. gastroenteritis

___7. peritonitis

___8. ulcers

a. infection of the peritoneum

b. inflammation of the appendix

c. inflammation of the gallbladder

d. inflammation of the stomach and intestines

e. open areas in the digestive system that may bleed

f. patient forces herself to vomit or uses laxatives to prevent nutrient absorption

g. patient refuses to eat because she thinks she is fat

h. rectum is filled with hard stool

Medical Terminology

Combine "gastr" with the following suffixes. Write the words and their meanings.

-ostomy _____

-ectomy_____

LANGUAGE AT WORK

Linda is a nursing assistant and Mrs. Chen is a patient with the disease diabetes mellitus.

Linda: Mrs. Chen, here's your lunch tray. May I see your identification bracelet while I check the name on the menu?

Mrs. Chen: OK, but I'm not sure that I'm really hungry.

Linda: Is there something wrong?

Mrs. Chen: No, I just don't feel like eating anything.

Linda: I'll take off the cover and we can see what there is. Chicken, mashed potatoes, and peas. That looks good! And there's some soup.

Mrs. Chen: Oh, I don't think I can eat anything.

Linda: It's important that you eat a little bit. Why don't you try some of the soup? I'll cover the chicken again until you're ready for it.

Mrs. Chen: All right, I'll try some soup.

Linda: Mrs. Chen, you ate about half of the soup. Do you think you could try a little chicken?

Mrs. Chen: No, I can't eat another bite. Please take the tray away.

Linda goes to the nurse.

Linda: Jane, Mrs. Chen only ate half a bowl of soup for lunch. She refused the rest of the food.

Continued on next page.

Jane: She hasn't been eating well recently. I'll go in and see her in a little while.

Linda: Meanwhile I'll keep a piece of fruit on her table in case she wants it later.

Questions

1. Why doesn't Mrs. Chen want her lunch?

_____

2. What does Mrs. Chen eat?

_____

3. How does Linda make sure Mrs. Chen is getting the right tray?

_____

4. What does Linda say to encourage Mrs. Chen to eat?

_____

5. What does Linda do when Mrs. Chen refuses to eat most of her meal?

_____

COMPETENCY CHECKLIST 35: GIVING THE PATIENT A TRAY

ACTIONS	SATISFACTORY	UNSATISFACTORY (COMMENTS)
Perform beginning procedure actions. Check menu and patient's nameband.		
Check menu with items on tray.		
For patient who can feed herself, assist with opening packets, cutting food, and removing covers.		
Give patient assistive devices. Place towel or chux over the chest.		
Never accept food from the tray.		
Remove overbed table and raise side rails. Perform ending procedure actions.		

INSTRUCTOR'S SIGNATURE _____ DATE _____

COMPETENCY CHECKLIST 36: FEEDING A PATIENT

ACTIONS	SATISFACTORY	UNSATISFACTORY (COMMENTS)
Perform beginning procedure actions. Set patient up for meal. Check nameband and tray.		
Explain foods to patient and ask what food to start with.		
Use tip of spoon, half full, to put food into the mouth. If weakness on one side of mouth, put food into strong side. Allow patient to swallow 1 mouthful before offering the next.		
Offer liquid after 2 or 3 mouthfuls. Do not use straws for hot liquids.		
Allow hot food to cool a little. Test temperature by using spoon to put drop of food on inside of your wrist. Perform ending procedure actions.		

INSTRUCTOR'S SIGNATURE _____ DATE _____

COMPETENCY CHECKLIST 37: CARING FOR A PATIENT WITH AN INTRAVENOUS TUBE

ACTIONS	SATISFACTORY	UNSATISFACTORY (COMMENTS)
Perform beginning procedure actions. Patient should not be lying on tubing. Observe IV site for redness, swelling, or pain and report to nurse.		
Do not take blood pressure on arm with IV.		
To remove gown, take off unaffected arm first, then off arm with IV. Cover patient with clean gown.		

COMPETENCY CHECKLIST 37: CARING FOR A PATIENT WITH AN INTRAVENOUS TUBE (CONTINUED)

ACTIONS	SATISFACTORY	UNSATISFACTORY (COMMENTS)
Work gown up over tubing. Take bag off IV pole and work gown over IV bag. Keep IV bag higher than IV site.		
Holding IV bag in your hand, put hand through sleeve of clean gown as if putting gown on your arm.		
Hang bag back on pole. Work gown over tubing and put it on arm with IV. Then put gown on unaffected arm.		
If IV is on a pump, do not disconnect it. Call the nurse.		
If IV tubing comes apart, put pressure on IV site (wear gloves) and call for help. Perform ending procedure actions.		

INSTRUCTOR'S SIGNATURE _____ DATE _____

COMPETENCY CHECKLIST 38: MEASURING AND RECORDING A PATIENT'S INTAKE

ACTIONS	SATISFACTORY	UNSATISFACTORY (COMMENTS)
Perform beginning procedure actions. Pour what is left of liquid into measuring cup and note the ccs. Subtract it from amount patient started with to get amount she drank.		
Record the amount she drank and the time. Total the numbers for the shift and for the entire day. Perform ending procedure actions.		

INSTRUCTOR'S SIGNATURE _____ DATE _____

COMPETENCY CHECKLIST 39: COLLECTING A STOOL SPECIMEN

ACTIONS	SATISFACTORY	UNSATISFACTORY (COMMENTS)
Perform beginning procedure actions. If patient uses bedpan or commode, make sure no urine enters pan or collection container.		
If patient uses toilet, position specimen pan under toilet seat.		
Wear gloves. Use wooden tongue depressors to transfer stool into sterile specimen container. Fill ⅓ to ½ full.		
Put label on container and place in plastic bag. Perform ending procedure actions.		

INSTRUCTOR'S SIGNATURE _____ DATE _____

COMPETENCY CHECKLIST 40: TESTING STOOL FOR OCCULT BLOOD

ACTIONS	SATISFACTORY	UNSATISFACTORY (COMMENTS)
Perform beginning procedure actions. Wear gloves. Obtain uncontaminated stool sample. Have ready test card, developing solution, and wooden stick.		
Use stick to take small amount of stool and put on left window on opened card. Take small amount from another area of stool and put it on right window.		

COMPETENCY CHECKLIST 40:
TESTING STOOL FOR OCCULT BLOOD (CONTINUED)

ACTIONS	SATISFACTORY	UNSATISFACTORY (COMMENTS)
Close cover, and open back panel. Place 1 drop of developing solution on each window and on control dots. Within a minute control dot will turn purple. If either or both windows turn purple, test is positive for blood. Report results to nurse. Perform ending procedure actions.		

INSTRUCTOR'S SIGNATURE _____ DATE _____

COMPETENCY CHECKLIST 41: GIVING AN ENEMA

ACTIONS	SATISFACTORY	UNSATISFACTORY (COMMENTS)
Perform beginning procedure actions. Fill enema container with warm 105°F water.		
Add liquid soap. Gently mix.		
Open clamp and allow some water to run through to remove air.		
Turn patient onto left side in Sims' position. Hang enema bag about 18 to 24 inches above mattress.		
Insert tube 2 to 4 inches into rectum. Open clamp and allow water to flow in until patient cannot hold any more. Position patient on bedpan. Report results to nurse. Perform ending procedure actions.		

INSTRUCTOR'S SIGNATURE _____ DATE _____

Chapter 14: Nutrition

VOCABULARY

agriculture	food pyramid	processed
amino acids	grain	saturated fat
artificial	habit	skim
balanced diet	ingredient	tradition
calories	linked	vegetarian
carbohydrate	malnourished	visible
clot	metabolism	vitamin
complex	mineral	whole milk
empty calorie	obesity	whole grain
essential	plaque	
financial	preservative	

WHAT IS GOOD NUTRITION?

Vocabulary Sentences

1. Everyone needs to eat a **balanced diet** for good health.
2. A complete protein contains all the **amino acids** needed by the body.
3. **Complex carbohydrates** can be found in **whole grains**.
4. Sweets are high in **empty calories**.
5. **Vitamins** and **minerals** are needed by the body for growth.
6. The base of the **food pyramid** is grains.
7. A person who makes poor food choices may be **malnourished**.

Label the Diagram

Label the sections of the food pyramid with the types of food and number of recommended servings, Figure 14–1.

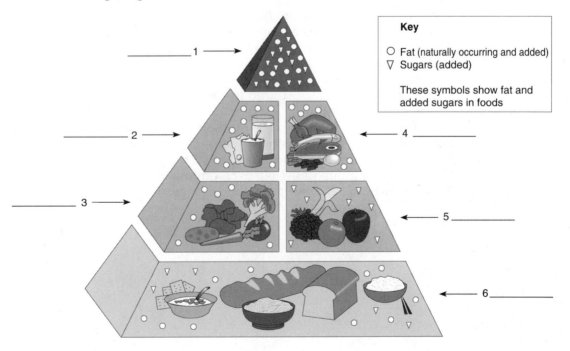

Figure 14–1

THE RELATIONSHIP BETWEEN FOOD AND HEALTH

Vocabulary Sentences

1. **Obesity** is a major health problem in the United States.
2. **Plaque** in the arteries can cause coronary artery disease.
3. The more active a person is the higher his **metabolism** will be.

Short Answer

List 6 diseases linked to poor eating habits.

1. _____
2. _____
3. _____
4. _____
5. _____
6. _____

READING LABELS

Vocabulary Sentences

1. We must rely on the nutrition labels of **processed** foods to tell us what nutrients are inside.
2. We should avoid foods high in **saturated fat**.
3. **Preservatives** and **artificial** flavors and colors are listed in the **ingredients** on food labels.

The Nutrition Crossword Puzzle

Across

4. Being very overweight
7. Not real; food items that are not found naturally
9. A nutrient that provides energy in simple or complex form
10. Food that is no longer in a whole, natural state
11. Having poor nutrition or an unhealthy diet
13. A substance that makes up proteins
15. A deposit of fatty material found inside arteries
16. Taking in and using food
17. Chemicals that are added to food to keep it fresh longer
19. Milk from which no fat has been removed
20. Milk products containing no fat
21. The habits of a group of people over a number of years
22. A person who does not eat meat, or a person who does not eat any animal products
23. Having to do with farming

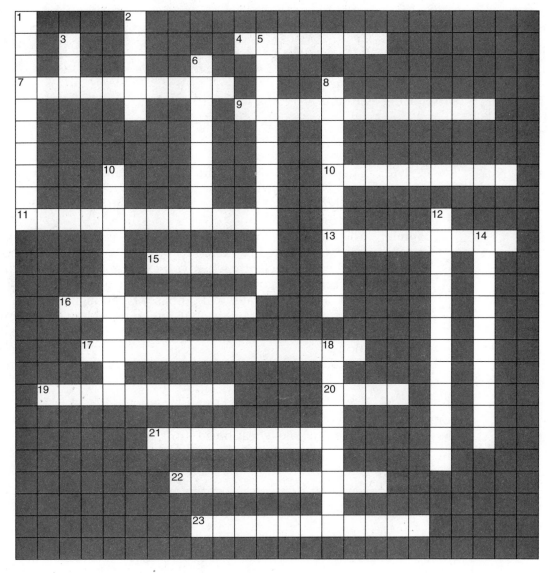

Figure 14–2

Down

1. Process by which nutrients are absorbed into blood and used by the cells
2. A plant containing cereal seeds, such as wheat, rice, corn and rye
3. An energy providing nutrient used by the body when carbohydrates are not available
5. Food containing all the nutrients needed by the body to be healthy
6. Units for measuring the amount of energy contained in a food
8. A picture of how to build a balanced diet based on the 4 food groups
10. A substance found in animal fats that is necessary to the cells. Too much can lead to heart disease.
12. The fat that comes from an animal source and contains more cholesterol than unsaturated fats
14. Individual food items that are contained in a packaged food
18. Absolutely necessary

LANGUAGE AT WORK

Two nursing assistants are going to lunch together.

Sylvia: Let's go down to the cafeteria for lunch. What do you feel like having?

Gerry: I think I'll have a hamburger and french fries and chocolate milk.

Sylvia: That sounds delicious, but I have to watch my calories. I'm trying to lose some weight.

Gerry: Really? I know I should lose some weight, too, but it's too hard to stay on a diet.

Sylvia: You know, I've lost 10 pounds already and it hasn't been too hard. I've started to exercise 3 or 4 times a week. Your body uses food more efficiently when you exercise. That salad with sliced chicken looks good. One slice of whole wheat bread, a piece of fruit, and some water will probably be enough.

Gerry: Well, maybe you're right, but I'm going to have the hamburger. Where do you exercise? That sounds like fun. Could I come along?

Sylvia: Of course. We'll meet after work and I'll show you where I go.

Questions

Compare the lunch of hamburger, french fries, and chocolate milk with the lunch of salad with chicken, whole wheat bread, fruit, and water.

1. Which probably has more calories? Which probably has more fat?

_____

2. Which parts of the food pyramid does each food fit into?

_____

_____

_____

_____

_____

_____

3. What does Sylvia do to help her lose weight?

_____

_____

_____

Chapter 15: Urinary System/Helping the Patient with Elimination

VOCABULARY

antiseptic	diuretic	renal failure
bathroom privileges	donor	retain
biopsy	dysuria	trauma
bladder	excrete	urea
catheterization	flank	ureter
circumcised	hematuria	urethra
clean-voided specimen	kidney	urinalysis
cloudy	kidney stones	urinary catheter
cystitis	leukocyte	urinary retention
cystoscopy	nephron	urinary sphincter
dialysis	potassium	urinary meatus
distinctive	recipient	void

ABBREVIATIONS

ac	before meals		**pc**	after meals
BID	twice a day or 2 times a day		**q2h**	every 2 hours
BRP	bathroom privileges		**q4h**	every 4 hours
CVS	clean-voided specimen		**qh**	every hour
daily	every day		**QID**	4 times a day
h	hour		**TID**	3 times a day
HS	at bedtime, when the patient goes to sleep		**U/A**	urinalysis
			UTI	urinary tract infection
IVP	intravenous pyelogram			

HOW THE URINARY SYSTEM EXCRETES WASTES

Vocabulary Sentences

1. The urinary system **retains** some substances and **excretes** others.
2. There are more than 1 million **nephrons** inside each **kidney**.
3. Urine contains water, salt, **urea**, and other waste products.
4. The ureters carry the urine from the kidneys to the **bladder**.
5. The **urinary sphincter** controls the flow of urine from the bladder into the **urethra**.
6. The **urinary meatus** is located in different places on men and women.

Label the Diagram

Label the parts of the urinary system on the diagram, Figure 15–1.

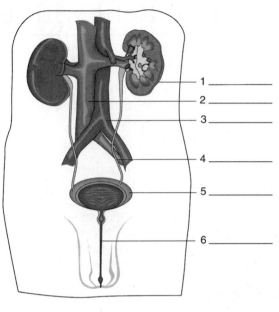

1 _____
2 _____
3 _____

4 _____

5 _____

6 _____

Figure 15–1

HELPING THE PATIENT WITH URINARY EXCRETION

Vocabulary Sentences

1. In the health care setting we often say **void** instead of urinate.
2. A patient taking **diuretics** needs to eat **potassium**-rich foods like oranges and bananas.
3. **Catheterization** is the process of inserting a **urinary catheter**.
4. A straight catheter may be used if a patient has **urinary retention**.

Discussion Questions

1. Name the 4 types of catheters and when each might be used.

_____

_____

_____

_____

Short Answer

Rewrite each of the following sentences using as many abbreviations as possible.

1. The registered nurse told the nursing assistant to check Mr. Overton's blood pressure every 4 hours.

   _____

   _____

2. The patient was incontinent of urine 2 times today.

   _____

   _____

3. The doctor ordered the patient to be ambulated 3 times a day.

   _____

   _____

4. The licensed practical nurse gives the patient his medication before meals.

   _____

   _____

5. Vital signs are often taken 4 times a day.

   _____

   _____

6. Ms. Clampton in the intensive care unit must be turned every 2 hours.

   _____

   _____

7. The patient with tuberculosis should have nourishment at bedtime.

   _____

   _____

8. As part of his bladder retraining program, Mr. Jones should be given the urinal every hour.

   _____

   _____

OBTAINING INFORMATION ABOUT URINE

Vocabulary Sentences

1. If a patient has **bathroom privileges** he may walk to toilet as needed.
2. A **urinalysis** checks to see if urine is clear or **cloudy**.
3. **Antiseptic** towelettes are used to clean the peri area before collecting a **clean-voided specimen**.
4. A multi-stix can be used to test the urine for **leukocytes**.

Short Answer

Output Section of Intake and Output Form

Time	Urine	Emesis	BM	Other/ Kind
8 Hour Total				
8 Hour Total				
8 Hour Total				
24 Hour Total				

Figure 15–2

Use the following measurements to fill out the urinary output portion of the I&O form, Figure 15–2.

0630 patient voided 450 ml urine
0900 patient voided 220 ml urine
1330 patient voided 345 ml urine
1615 patient voided 280 ml urine
2220 patient voided 370 ml urine

Role Play

Choose a nursing assistant, nurse, and patient for this role play. The nurse asks the nursing assistant to get a clean-voided specimen from the patient and bring it to her so it can be sent to the lab. The nursing assistant goes to the patient and explains what the patient must do. When the nursing assistant has the specimen, she returns to the nurse and gives report. You may use the following sentence to get you started or use your own.

Nurse: Jane, please get a CVS from Ms. Periello and bring it to me. We need to get it to the lab stat.

CONDITIONS AND DISEASES

Vocabulary Sentences

1. **Dysuria** and **hematuria** are symptoms of a urinary tract infection.
2. **Cystitis** is a urinary tract infection.
3. **Cystoscopy** and a **biopsy** can be done to diagnose bladder cancer.
4. **Renal failure** can be treated with **dialysis**.
5. A person who donates an organ is called a **donor** and a person who receives an organ is called a **recipient**.

Discussion Question

1. Why is cystitis more common in women than men and what can they do to prevent it?

   _____

   _____

   _____

   _____

Short Answer

1. "Ur" is the word root for urine. How many words can you find in this chapter with "ur" as the root? List them below.

   _____

   _____

   _____

2. "Dys" is the prefix meaning difficult or painful. Break down the following word into its parts and write the meaning of each.

   dysuria _____

3. Hematuria means blood in the urine. What does the prefix "hemat" mean?

   _____

The word root "cysto" means bladder. What is the meaning of the following 2 words?

4. cystitis _____

5. cystoscopy _____

6. The word root "nephro" means kidneys. What does "nephritis" mean?

   _____

Renal is another word used to refer to the kidneys. Below are 3 vocabulary terms that use renal. Write the meaning of each.

7. renal failure _____

8. renal transplant _____

9. renal calculi _____

LANGUAGE AT WORK

Carmen, a nursing assistant, talks to Mr. Feinberg about bladder retraining after he has had a catheter removed.

Carmen: Mr. Feinberg, how do you feel now that the nurse has taken out your catheter?

Mr. Feinberg: I'm glad to have it out, but I feel nervous about "having an accident."

Carmen: I can understand that you feel that way. We plan to help you as much as we can. First of all, here is a urinal. I'll place it on your bedside table where you can reach it as soon as you feel the need to urinate.

Mr. Feinberg: I suppose I can try.

Carmen: Good. I'll be back to check on you in an hour to see if you'd like to get up and walk to the bathroom. If you need me sooner, here's the call button.

Questions

1. What does Mr. Feinberg mean when he says that he is nervous about "having an accident"?

_____

2. What does Carmen do to help Mr. Feinberg?

_____

3. How do you think Mr. Feinberg feels about having the catheter removed? Why?

_____

_____

4. Why is it important for Carmen to be especially understanding and helpful in this situation?

_____

_____

COMPETENCY CHECKLIST 42: GIVING CATHETER CARE

ACTIONS	SATISFACTORY	UNSATISFACTORY (COMMENTS)
Perform beginning procedure actions. Wear gloves. Give peri care using downward strokes away from urinary meatus along catheter for 3 to 4 inches.		
Secure catheter to thigh with Velcro strap.		
Tape may be used if strap is not available.		
Take drain out of holder. Clean it with alcohol prep and open clamp.		
Drain urine into patient's own specimen pan. Do not allow drain to touch anything.		
Clean drain with another alcohol prep and return it to holder.		
Note amount, color, and odor of urine. Report anything unusual. Empty pan and wash it out.		
A leg drainage bag is held on by adjustable straps. The drain valve on bottom can be turned to open.		
To change drainage bags, disconnect tubing from catheter and cover end with protector. Connect new bag. Protect bed with chux. Perform ending procedure actions.		

INSTRUCTOR'S SIGNATURE _____ DATE _____

COMPETENCY CHECKLIST 43:
MEASURING AND RECORDING A PATIENT'S OUTPUT

ACTIONS	SATISFACTORY	UNSATISFACTORY (COMMENTS)
Perform beginning procedure actions. Wear gloves. Pour urine from bedpan into measuring container. Make sure no toilet tissue has been put into bedpan.		
If urine is already in specimen pan or urinal, hold it at eye level or put it on a level surface and read number of ccs. Remember the number or write it on a piece of paper.		
Empty urine into toilet and rinse out pan.		
After removing gloves and washing hands, record ccs under the urine column of the Intake and Output form. Vomitus is measured and recorded under emesis column. Loose, watery stool is recorded under BM. Perform ending procedure actions.		

INSTRUCTOR'S SIGNATURE _____ DATE _____

COMPETENCY CHECKLIST 44: COLLECTING A URINE SPECIMEN

ACTIONS	SATISFACTORY	UNSATISFACTORY (COMMENTS)
Perform beginning procedure actions. Wear gloves. If patient has gone to the bathroom, accept the container.		
Set container on paper towel and label it immediately. Make sure urine from bedpan, urinal or commode is not contaminated. Pour urine into container in bathroom or dirty utility room. Label it immediately.		
Place container in plastic bag. Have specimen and paperwork transported to lab.		
Store in specimen refrigerator if necessary.		
To obtain urine from an indwelling catheter, coil catheter so urine collects. Wipe port with alcohol.		
Using a sterile needle and 20 cc syringe, withdraw at least 20 cc of urine and put it into sterile container. Label container. Dispose of needle in sharps container. Perform ending procedure actions.		

INSTRUCTOR'S SIGNATURE _____ DATE _____

COMPETENCY CHECKLIST 45:
COLLECTING A CLEAN-VOIDED URINE SPECIMEN

ACTIONS	SATISFACTORY	UNSATISFACTORY (COMMENTS)
Perform beginning procedure actions. Wear gloves. Peri care is given with soap and water or with antiseptic towelettes. For a male, have patient void into urinal, stop the flow and then catch some urine in the sterile container.		
For a female, after peri care, position patient on bedpan. After she voids a little, catch some in the sterile container.		
If the patient uses the bathroom, give instructions on what to do. Perform ending procedure actions.		

INSTRUCTOR'S SIGNATURE _____ DATE _____

Chapter 16: Endocrine System/Patient with Diabetes Mellitus

VOCABULARY

acidic
acute hypoglycemic reaction
athlete
complication
diabetes mellitus
diabetic ketoacidosis
efficient
equivalent
estrogen
fatigue
fight or flight reaction
glucagon
glucose
glucose tolerance test

goiter
hormone
hyperglycemia
hypoglycemia
hypoglycemic
insulin-dependent
insulin
ketone
Kussmaul respirations
level of consciousness
menstruation
mild
monitoring
neuropathy
non–insulin-dependent

ovary
polydipsia
polyphagia
polyuria
progesterone
puberty
pubic
scrotum
secrete
side effect
steroid
subcutaneous
testosterone
testis
thyroid

ABBREVIATIONS

ADA	American Diabetes Association	**LOC**	level of consciousness
DKA	diabetic ketoacidosis	**NIDDM**	non–insulin-dependent diabetes mellitus
DM	diabetes mellitus		
GTT	glucose tolerance test	**S&A**	sugar and acetone
IDDM	insulin-dependent diabetes mellitus	**SC**	subcutaneously

HOW THE ENDOCRINE SYSTEM CONTROLS BODY FUNCTIONS

Vocabulary Sentences

1. Endocrine glands **secrete** hormones.
2. The **thyroid** is located around the trachea.
3. **Steroids** are hormones that are necessary for life.
4. The **testes** are inside the **scrotum**.
5. At **puberty** the **ovaries** begin to secrete **estrogen** and **progesterone**, which cause **menstruation**.
6. The pancreas produces **insulin** and **glucagon**.

Content:

Label the Diagram

Label the parts of the endocrine system on the diagram, Figure 16–1.

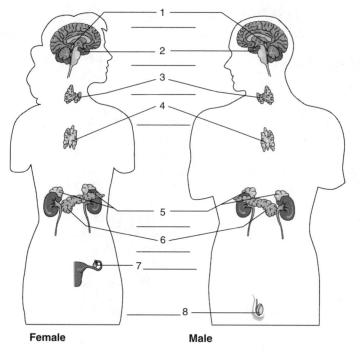

Female   Male

Figure 16–1

DIABETES MELLITUS

Vocabulary Sentences

1. The two types of **diabetes mellitus** are **insulin-dependent diabetes mellitus** and **non–insulin-dependent diabetes mellitus**.
2. Three common symptoms of IDDM are **polyuria, polydipsia,** and **polyphagia**.
3. Some patients with NIDDM take oral **hypoglycemic** medication.
4. The **glucose tolerance test** is used to diagnose diabetes.
5. **Hypoglycemia** and **hyperglycemia** are 2 conditions diabetics must avoid.
6. The **ADA** diet lists foods that are equivalent to one another, so that diabetics can make good food choices.
7. Insulin injections are given by **subcutaneous** injection.
8. By **monitoring** the blood glucose level, diabetics know how much insulin to take.
9. One **complication** of diabetes is **acute hypoglycemic reaction**.
10. **Kussmaul respirations** are 1 symptom of **diabetic ketoacidosis**.
11. A nursing assistant must observe the patient for any change in the **level of consciousness**.

Discussion Questions

1. Why is the nursing assistant's role so important in the care of diabetic patients?

2. Review the 5 things nursing assistants need to remember when caring for a diabetic patient.

Role Play

Choose 2 nursing assistants for this role play. The nursing assistants meet in the nurses' station. The first nursing assistant has a diabetic patient to care for. The second nursing assistant is new and has not had a diabetic patient to care for. The first nursing assistant explains what to watch for and what to do for a diabetic patient. The second asks questions about caring for a diabetic patient. (For helpful words and phrases to use in this role play refer to the Language at Work at the end of this chapter.)

OTHER CONDITIONS AND DISEASES

Vocabulary Sentences

1. A **goiter** occurs when the thyroid gland enlarges.
2. The use of steroids by **athletes** has many dangerous **side effects**.

Medical Terminology

The following prefixes are used several times in this chapter:

hyper above or more than normal
hypo   below or less than normal
poly   many; more than normal

Combine the prefixes above with the following word parts to get the names of the conditions and diseases defined below. Write the name of the condition or disease in the space next to the definition.

thyroidism
glycemia
uria
dipsia
phagia

_____ 1. abnormal thirst

_____ 2. low blood sugar

_____ 3. abnormal hunger

_____ 4. a disease caused by too much thyroid hormone being produced

_____ 5. abnormal urine production

_____ 6. a disease caused by too little thyroid hormone being produced

_____ 7. high blood sugar

Based on the exercise you have just completed, list the word roots for:

_____ hunger

_____ thirst

_____ urine production

Discussion Question

1. Some professional athletes and teenage athletes use steroid drugs to build up their strength. Why do you think they do something that is dangerous to their health? What does this say about our culture and sports?

LANGUAGE AT WORK

Sandy: One of my patients is a diabetic.
Ralph: Oh, really? One of my patients has diabetes also.
Sandy: Is your patient insulin dependent?
Ralph: No, he's non–insulin-dependent.
Sandy: Oh, mine is insulin dependent. Diabetics really need special care, especially for their feet.
Ralph: You're right. I checked my patient's feet this morning to make sure that there were no red or open areas.
Sandy: What about the diet? It's hard for my patient to keep away from sweets. All her life she was used to eating candy and cake. Now she's taking insulin and is on a 1800 calorie ADA diet. Actually, she's doing very well. The nurse is teaching her how to give herself insulin shots and to test her blood glucose level.
Ralph: My patient is also doing well. If he stays on his diet and exercises, he might not even need to take any pills. Well, talk to you later.

Questions

1. Who has a non–insulin-dependent patient?

_____

2. Why does Ralph need to check his patient's feet?

_____

3. What kind of diet is Sandy's patient on?

_____

4. What is the nurse teaching Sandy's patient to do?

_____

Chapter 17: Nervous System/Understanding the Brain and the Senses

VOCABULARY

aphasia
brain dead
brain stem
cataracts
central nervous system
cerebellum
cerebrospinal fluid
cerebrum
conjunctiva
conjunctivitis
conscious
cornea
corrective
degenerative
encephalitis
epilepsy
eustachian tube
gag
general seizure

glaucoma
hemisphere
hemorrhage
iris
laser
legally blind
lens
lumbar puncture
magnify
meninges
meningitis
motor nerve
multiple sclerosis
nerve
neurologic
neuron
olfactory cell
otitis media
Parkinson's disease

partial seizure
pinna
postictal
pupil
receptor
reflex
respirator
retina
sclera
seizure
sensory nerve
slurred speech
taste bud
transient ischemic
    attack
tremor
tympanic membrane
visual acuity

ABBREVIATIONS

c	with	OD	right eye
C	correction	OS	left eye
CNS	central nervous system	OU	both eyes
CT	computerized tomography	PNS	peripheral nervous system
EEG	electroencephalogram	s	without
LP	lumbar puncture	TIA	transient ischemic attack
MRI	magnetic resonance imaging	VA	visual acuity
MS	multiple sclerosis		

THE NERVOUS SYSTEM AS A CONTROL AND COMMUNICATION SYSTEM

Vocabulary Sentences

1. **Neurons** connect together to form a **nerve**.
2. **Motor nerves** tell your hand to turn the pages of a book and your eyes to follow the words on the page.
3. **Sensory nerves** carry sight messages to your brain so you can read the words.
4. The **central nervous system** is made up of the brain and the spinal cord.
5. The **meninges** protect and nourish the brain.
6. **Cerebrospinal fluid** carries nutrients and wastes between the brain cells and the blood.
7. The **cerebrum** is divided into 2 **hemispheres**.
8. He was still **conscious** when they brought him into the emergency department.
9. The **cerebellum** has control over the skeletal muscles.

10. A **reflex** is an automatic reaction of the body that is not under conscious control.
11. When a light is shined on 1 **pupil** both pupils should get smaller.
12. When the tongue depressor is placed on the back of the tongue, the patient will **gag**.

Label the Diagram

Label the parts of the nervous system in the diagram, Figure 17–1.

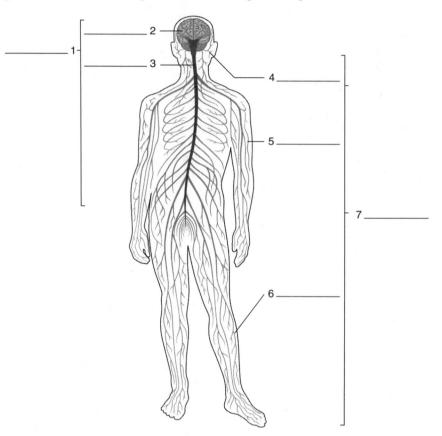

Figure 17–1

Listening

Circle the word you hear.

1. cerebrum	cerebellum	cranial
2. neuron	nerve	nervous
3. parental	peripheral	perineum
4. sensory	central	system
5. conscious	unconscious	consciously

THE SENSORY ORGANS

Vocabulary Sentences

1. The **conjunctiva** lines the inside of the eyelids and covers the eyeball.
2. The **sclera** is the white of the eye and the **iris** is the colored part.
3. The **cornea** covers the front of the eye.
4. When the **lens** does not change shape correctly, a person needs glasses with **corrective** lenses.
5. In the **retina** the messages of what you see are sent to the brain.

6. An eye chart is a quick way to check a patient's **visual acuity**.
7. Another name for the **tympanic membrane** is the eardrum.
8. The **eustachian tubes** allow air pressure to become stable within the ear.
9. Hearing aids help **magnify** sounds.
10. Some areas of the body are more sensitive to touch because they have more **receptors**.

Label the Diagrams

Label the parts of the eye and ear in the diagrams, Figures 17–2 and 17–3.

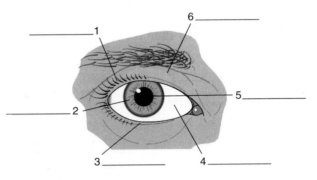

Figure 17–2

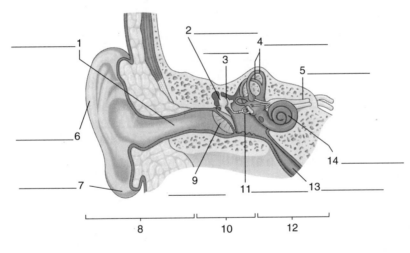

Figure 17–3

Categorize

Categorize the items in the list below as part of the brain, eye or ear.

auditory canal
brain stem
cerebellum
cerebrospinal fluid
cerebrum
cochlea
conjunctiva

cornea
eustachian tubes
iris
lacrimal gland
lens
meninges

pinna
retina
sclera
semicircular canals
tympanic membrane
ventricles

Brain

_____

_____

_____

_____

_____

_____

Eye

_____

_____

_____

_____

_____

_____

Ear

_____

_____

_____

_____

_____

_____

CONDITIONS AND DISEASES

Vocabulary Sentences

1. One cause of a cerebrovascular accident can be a **hemorrhage**.
2. Mr. Ilia has **aphasia** so you must look at him directly when communicating with him.
3. Mrs. Flenner had a **TIA**, so the doctor told her about some things she can do to try to prevent a CVA.
4. Patients with **Parkinson's disease** may have hand **tremors**.
5. A **seizure** disorder is sometimes called epilepsy.
6. A **partial** seizure can be so mild that it is not even noticed.
7. Mr. Jones had a **general seizure** this morning so he will need **postictal** care.

8. The **EEG** is used to find out if a patient is **brain dead**.
9. Miss Connor was put on a **respirator** this afternoon.
10. The **CT scan** and **MRI** allow the doctor to see inside the skull and brain.
11. **Meningitis** and **encephalitis** can cause permanent **neurologic** damage.
12. Good hand washing is important to keep **conjunctivitis** from spreading.
13. Mr. Bashir had **cataract** surgery so please watch for severe pain, nausea, or vomiting.
14. **Glaucoma** may be treated with **laser** therapy.
15. **Otitis media** is common in children because of their shorter eustachian tubes.

Writing

Write a paragraph describing what you would do for a patient who has just had a seizure.

_____

_____

_____

_____

_____

_____

_____

Role Play

For this role play choose a nurse, a nursing assistant, and a head trauma patient. The nursing assistant is caring for a patient with head trauma. The nurse asks the nursing assistant to check the patient's level of consciousness when taking vital signs and to report anything unusual to the nurse right away. The nursing assistant takes the vital signs, checks the level of consciousness, and reports back.

Medical Terminology

Match the 2 halves of the sentences. Then circle the word parts that mean brain, half, hearing, vision, and ball.

___ 1. The auditory nerve

___ 2. The optic nerve

___ 3. Hemiplegia

___ 4. A cerebrovascular accident

___ 5. An electroencephalogram

___ 6. Encephalitis

___ 7. A hemisphere

___ 8. Cerebrospinal fluid

a. is an inflammation of the brain.
b. sends vision messages to the brain.
c. is half of ball.
d. protects and nourishes the brain and spinal cord.
e. measures the electrical brain activity.
f. sends hearing messages to the brain.
g. affects half of the body.
h. happens when blood has a problem reaching the brain.

List two word roots that refer to the brain.

1. _____

2. _____

LANGUAGE AT WORK

Joe:	Hello, Mrs. Merullo. The nurse asked me to test your eyes. Do you wear glasses for distance?
Mrs. Merullo:	Yes, I do. Should I put them on?
Joe:	Yes, please. Stand right over here and put your feet at this line on the floor. Cover your left eye and read the line with the smallest letters you can see clearly.
Mrs. Merullo:	I can read line number 7. F,E,L,O,R,Z,P.

Note by looking at Figure 17–11 that Mrs. Merullo read 2 letters wrong. If she only read 1 letter wrong, you could write that her vision was 20/25 [–1] in the right eye but since she missed 2 she must read the next line up.

Joe:	Mrs. Merullo, try reading line number 6.
Mrs. Merullo:	E,D,F,C,Z,P.
Joe:	Good, now cover your right eye and read the line with the smallest letters you can see clearly.
Mrs. Merullo:	Line 7. F,E,L,O,P,Z,D.

Questions

1. How would Joe record Mrs. Merullo's vision using the abbreviations learned in this chapter?

   _____

2. Write out in words the following visual acuity: VA s C: OD 20/50, OS 20/40.

   _____

3. Write out in words the following: OS 20/20 [–1.]

   _____

COMPETENCY CHECKLIST 46: CARING FOR A PATIENT WITH SEIZURES

ACTIONS	SATISFACTORY	UNSATISFACTORY (COMMENTS)
Assist patient to floor. Place something soft under head, loosen clothing around neck. Call for help and stay with patient.		
Turn patient onto side, if possible.		
Clear area of furniture. Maintain privacy, if possible.		
Observe seizure. Do not try to restrain patient or put anything into mouth. Note length of time of seizure and report.		

INSTRUCTOR'S SIGNATURE _____ DATE _____

Chapter 18: Reproductive System/ Human Sexuality

VOCABULARY

abstinent
amniotic sac
birth control
cervix
cesarean section
characteristic
chlamydia
chromosome
contraception
dominant gene
dysfunctional
ectopic pregnancy
ejaculation
embryo
endometriosis
epididymis
erection
fertilization
fetus
fibroid
follicle
fraternal twin
gene

gonorrhea
hemorrhoid
hot flash
hysterectomy
identical twin
immature
implanted
infertility
insomnia
labor
mammary gland
mammogram
mastectomy
menarche
menstrual cycle
miscarriage
oviduct
ovulation
pair
Pap smear
pelvic inflammatory
    disease
placenta

prenatal
prostate gland
recessive gene
seminiferous tubule
sexually transmitted
    disease
sitz bath
spontaneous abortion
syphilis
tampon
testicle
toxemia
ultrasound
umbilical cord
uterus
vagina
vaginal irrigation
vaginitis
vas deferens
virginity
vulva
zygote

ABBREVIATIONS

C section	cesarean section	**PSA**	prostate-specific antigen
D&C	dilation and curettage	**STD**	sexually transmitted disease
ERT	estrogen replacement therapy	**TURP**	transurethral resection of the prostate
PID	pelvic inflammatory disease	**US**	ultrasound

THE MALE REPRODUCTIVE SYSTEM

Vocabulary Sentences

1. Another name for the testes is **testicles**.
2. The **vas deferens** carries the sperm from the **epididymis** to the urethra during **ejaculation**.
3. The **prostate gland** adds fluid to the sperm to help make semen.
4. When the penis fills with blood, it is called an **erection**.

Label the Diagram

Label the parts of the male reproductive system on the diagram, Figure 18–1.

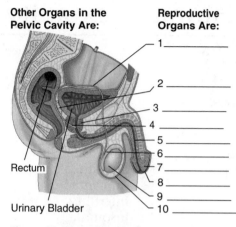

Other Organs in the Pelvic Cavity Are:

Reproductive Organs Are:

1 _____
2 _____
3 _____
4 _____
5 _____
6 _____
7 _____
8 _____
9 _____
10 _____

Rectum

Urinary Bladder

Figure 18–1

THE FEMALE REPRODUCTIVE SYSTEM

Vocabulary Sentences

1. Within the **ovary**, each **immature** egg is inside a **follicle**.
2. **Menarche** is the time of the first menstruation.
3. After **ovulation** the egg travels down the **oviduct** to the uterus.
4. The **cervix** opens up to allow a baby to be born through the **vagina**.
5. The external genitals of a woman are called the **vulva**.
6. Although the hymen is considered a sign of **virginity**, it can be broken in nonsexual ways.
7. The **mammary glands** produce milk after childbirth and play a role in sexuality.
8. The **menstrual** cycle prepares an egg for **fertilization**.
9. A sitz bath may be used as a treatment for **hemorrhoids**.

Label the Diagram

Label the parts of the female reproductive system on the diagrams, Figure 18–2.

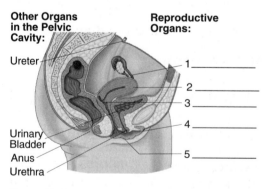

Other Organs in the Pelvic Cavity:

Reproductive Organs:

Ureter

1 _____
2 _____
3 _____
4 _____
5 _____

Urinary Bladder

Anus

Urethra

Figure 18–2

Medical Terminology

Find 3 words from this section that use the word root "ov" meaning "egg." Write the words and their definitions below.

1. _____

2. _____

3. _____

Find 3 words from this section that use the word root "men" meaning "month." Write the words and their definitions below.

1. _____

2. _____

3. _____

HOW HUMAN BEINGS REPRODUCE

Vocabulary Sentences

1. The **zygote** travels down the oviduct to the uterus where it is **implanted** and becomes an **embryo**.
2. The **fetus** floats in fluid inside the **amniotic sac**.
3. The **umbilical cord** attaches the embryo to the placenta.
4. When a pregnant woman goes into **labor**, she knows her baby is ready to be born.
5. A genetic disease is one that is passed on from parent to child in the **genes**.
6. The **chromosomes** of the mother and father combine to produce a child with **characteristics** of both.
7. Genes are either **dominant** or **recessive**.

Listening

One word in each sentence is **WRONG**. Listen to each sentence being read using the correct word. Circle the word that you hear that is different from what is written. Write the correct word on the line before the sentence.

_____ 1. The penis is the most visible part of the female reproductive system.

_____ 2. The vagina is about the size and shape of a pear and provides a place for a baby to grow.

_____ 3. The male reproductive system predicts testosterone.

_____ 4. The female reproductive symptom produces progesterone and estrogen.

_____ 5. Prenatal care is an extremely important factory in having a healthy baby.

_____ 6. The sperm and egg cells only have 23 chromosomes each so that when they combine they will have 146.

_____ 7. Genes carries hereditary diseases.

_____ 8. It is the egg cell of the father that determines the sex of the child.

HUMAN SEXUALITY

Vocabulary Sentences

1. All people must decide whether to have sex or remain **abstinent**.
2. Different methods of **birth control** can prevent pregnancy.
3. Lack of estrogen can cause women to suffer from **hot flashes** and **insomnia**.

Culture Exchange

Answer the following questions by yourself or with others from your birth country. Then share your answers with other cultural groups in your class.

1. How do people in your birth country learn about sex? Who teaches them?

   _____

2. At what age do people usually learn about sex?

   _____

3. At what age is a woman considered old enough to become a mother?

   _____

4. At what age is a man considered old enough to be a father?

   _____

5. How is an unmarried mother viewed in your culture?

   _____

6. How is a woman without children viewed in your culture?

   _____

7. How is a man without children viewed in your culture?

   _____

8. How is the use of contraception viewed in your culture?

   _____

9. What do you think of sex in the American culture?

   _____

After the culture exchange of information, answer the following questions.

1. What differences did you learn about how sex and sexuality are viewed by others in your class?

   _____

   _____

2. You may have patients with any of the sexual attitudes you heard from your classmates. You may also have patients with other sexual attitudes that seem strange or even wrong to you. What is expected of you as a nursing assistant in these situations?

   _____

   _____

CONDITIONS AND DISEASES

Vocabulary Sentences

1. A **mammogram** can detect breast cancer in the early stages when it can be cured.
2. Cervical cancer can be detected by a yearly **Pap smear**.
3. Mrs. Jimenez had a **hysterectomy**, but she still has her ovaries.
4. Two causes of **dysfunctional** uterine bleeding are **fibroids** and **endometriosis**.
5. When a couple is unable to conceive children they may see an **infertility** specialist.
6. A **D&C** was done by the doctor to diagnose the problem with the patient's uterus.
7. A **spontaneous abortion** is often called a **miscarriage**.
8. Ms. Nyguen has **toxemia** of pregnancy so she must eat a low-salt diet.
9. Often when there is a problem with a pregnancy or birth a **cesarean section** is done.
10. An **ultrasound** is used to check on the fetus inside the mother.
11. **Pelvic inflammatory disease** can be caused by sexually transmitted diseases.
12. Mr. Hernandez had a **TURP** on Wednesday.
13. **Gonorrhea** and **chlamydia** are common **STDs**.
14. **Syphilis** causes birth defects in babies.

Role Play

Choose a nurse, nursing assistant, and a patient for this role play. The nurse explains to the nursing assistant that there is a new mother on the floor with syphilis. Her baby was delivered by cesarean section and has birth defects. The nursing assistant will be caring for this patient.

Part 1
The nursing assistant goes to the patient to help her with morning care. The patient is rude and acts like she does not need anything from anybody.

Part 2
Later in the morning the nursing assistant is told to ask the patient if she wants to go to the nursery to see her baby. The patient does not want to see the baby and is rude to the nursing assistant again. The nursing assistant reports to the nurse.

Short Answer

1. Name 3 complications of pregnancy discussed in this chapter.

    1. _____
    2. _____
    3. _____

2. List 5 sexually transmitted diseases, their symptoms, and their treatments.

Disease	Symptoms	Treatment
1.		
2.		
3.		
4.		
5.		

LANGUAGE AT WORK

A conversation between a patient and a nursing assistant at a clinic.

Patient: I think I might be pregnant. I missed my period.

NA: What was the date that your last menstrual period started?

Patient: Let me think. Do you have a calendar? Oh yes, it was July 19th.

NA: That's almost 2 months ago. Did you want to make an appointment with the doctor?

Patient: Well, can't I just have a pregnancy test?

NA: It's important that you have an exam, too. If you are pregnant, prenatal care should be started as soon as possible. I can give you an appointment with Dr. Simon tomorrow at 3 PM.

Questions

1. What does the patient want from the nursing assistant?

   _____

2. Why does the nursing assistant say the patient must see the doctor?

   _____

COMPETENCY CHECKLIST 47:
SETTING UP FOR A PELVIC EXAMINATION

ACTIONS	SATISFACTORY	UNSATISFACTORY (COMMENTS)
Perform beginning procedure actions. Explain procedure to patient. Place feet in stirrups and drape so only perineum is exposed.		
Wear gloves. Prepare culture swabs as needed. Help patient off table. Perform ending procedure actions.		

INSTRUCTOR'S SIGNATURE _____ DATE _____

COMPETENCY CHECKLIST 48: GIVING A VAGINAL IRRIGATION

ACTIONS	SATISFACTORY	UNSATISFACTORY (COMMENTS)
Perform beginning procedure actions. Wear gloves. Have patient void. Place patient on clean bedpan in flat or semi-Fowler's position.		
Let small amount of solution flow over vulva.		
Insert tube 3 to 4 inches into vagina and let solution flow in. Rotate tube slightly. Stop flow if patient has discomfort and inform nurse.		
Place patient in sitting position on bedpan so solution can drain out. Perform ending procedure actions.		

INSTRUCTOR'S SIGNATURE _____ DATE _____

COMPETENCY CHECKLIST 49: GIVING A SITZ BATH

ACTIONS	SATISFACTORY	UNSATISFACTORY (COMMENTS)
Perform beginning procedure actions. Fill pan with warm water, and place under toilet seat with drainage holes toward the back.		
Hang prepared bag with 120° F water on hook near toilet. Have patient sit on toilet. Make sure patient is warm enough.		
Place tubing of bag into opening at front of pan. As water in pan cools, open clamp and let warm water flow into pan. Disinfect pan and return to patient's bedside table. Perform ending procedure actions.		

INSTRUCTOR'S SIGNATURE _____ DATE _____

Chapter 19: Patients with Special Needs/Caring for Surgical, Cancer and Dying Patients

VOCABULARY

antiembolism stockings
body image
chemotherapy
Cheyne-Stokes
    respirations
consent form
deceased
disfiguring
general anesthesia

grief
grimacing
immunotherapy
incentive spirometer
incision
mandatory
oncology
operative site
overdose

pneumatic boots
postmortem care
pulse oximeter
radiation
reconstructive
sterile field
syncope
terminal illness

ABBREVIATIONS

PCA pump   patient-controlled
                        analgesia pump

THE PATIENT WHO HAS SURGERY

Vocabulary Sentences

1. Patients must read, understand, and sign a **consent form** before having surgery.
2. Be sure to scrub Ms. Donnely's **operative site** with iodine solution.
3. The **pulse oximeter** measures the oxygen level of the blood.
4. A patient who has had **general anesthesia** should have an emesis basin nearby in case he vomits.
5. Mrs. Chung had **spinal anesthesia** so be sure she is kept lying flat.
6. The nursing assistant reported that the patient's vital signs were **stable**.
7. Ms. El Jafar states that she is in pain and I observed her **grimacing** and holding the siderail tightly.
8. Last night a drug **overdose** victim was brought in.
9. Ms. Del Greco's **incision** is healing well.
10. The **incentive spirometer** is helping Mr. Gonzalez to breathe deeply.
11. **Antiembolism stockings** squeeze the leg veins to aid circulation.
12. It is important to remember the difference between sterile and clean when setting up a **sterile field**.

Role Play

Choose a nursing assistant, a nurse, and a patient for this role play.

Part 1
The nurse orders the nursing assistant to take vital signs and make sure a patient is ready for surgery. The nursing assistant goes to the room and finds the patient looking out the window with a worried expression. When the nursing assistant comes in, the patient begins asking questions about the surgery and what happens afterward. The nursing assistant talks to the patient for a few minutes, makes sure the patient is physically ready for surgery, and then reports to the nurse about what happened.

Part 2

The nurse assigns the nursing assistant to prepare the room for the postop patient. The nursing assistant does this. The patient returns from surgery and is still sleepy from the general anesthesia. The nurse makes the first postop check and then gives the nursing assistant orders on what to do for the patient.

Part 3

Pick 1 emergency situation. A nursing assistant finds the patient in this situation. Explain what actions the nursing assistant takes. Then the nursing assistant gives report to the nurse.

THE CANCER PATIENT

Vocabulary Sentences

1. The study of cancer is called **oncology**.
2. **Chemotherapy, radiation** therapy, and **immunotherapy** are 3 types of cancer treatments.
3. Mrs. Beck had **disfiguring** cancer surgery and is having trouble accepting her changed **body image**.
4. Mrs. Beck is scheduled to have **reconstructive** breast surgery.

Writing

Write a paragraph explaining the special care cancer patients may need from a nursing assistant.

_____

_____

_____

_____

_____

_____

_____

THE PATIENT WITH A TERMINAL ILLNESS

Vocabulary Sentences

1. When a patient has a **terminal illness**, she and her family and friends will experience different stages of **grief**.
2. Mr. White is having **Cheyne-Stokes respirations**. Please tell his son to come in now.
3. The **deceased** will be taken to the morgue.

Short Answer

List the five stages of grief.

1. _____

2. _____

3. _____

4. _____

5. _____

Culture Exchange

Answer the following questions alone or with others from your birth country. When you are finished, share your answers with the rest of the class.

1. Who does the postmortem care in your birth country? What is done for postmortem care?

   _____

   _____

2. Where is the body taken after death?

   _____

   _____

3. What do people do to mark the end of someone's life? Do they gather together to honor the deceased in some way?

   _____

   _____

4. What happens to the body after the funeral?

   _____

   _____

5. What kind of support does the family of the deceased receive in the coming year?

   _____

   _____

After hearing the answers of your classmates, list the similarities between the way death is handled in your country and all the other countries you have just learned about.

_____

_____

Medical Terminology

Combine the word parts listed below to make words to fit the definitions listed.

pre-   before
post-   after
-op   operation
-mortem   death

_____ before the operation

_____ after death

_____ after the operation

"Pre" is a common prefix in English. List 3 other words where "pre" is used to mean "before." (You may use a dictionary.)

_____

_____

_____

LANGUAGE AT WORK

A conversation between 2 nursing assistants at a nursing home.

Manuel: Is Mrs. Holloway doing any better today?

Ev: Oh, you don't know yet! Mrs. Holloway is deceased.

Manuel: That's too bad. When did it happen?

Ev: She expired at about 3 am.

Manuel: Her daughter must feel awful. Was she with her mother when she passed away?

Ev: Yes, she was. Mrs. Holloway started to have Cheyne-Stokes respirations at about midnight and the nurse called her daughter and asked her if she wanted to come in. She arrived half an hour later.

Questions

1. Who is deceased? When did she die?

_____

2. Why did the nurse call Mrs. Holloway's daughter?

_____

3. List 2 ways to say that a person has died that are used in this conversation.

_____

COMPETENCY CHECKLIST 50: APPLYING ANTIEMBOLISM STOCKINGS

ACTIONS	SATISFACTORY	UNSATISFACTORY (COMMENTS)
Perform beginning procedure actions. Put your arm into stocking, grasp heel, and pull inside out.		
Place patient's toes into toes of stocking and gather stocking between your fingers.		
Place patient's heel into heel of stocking. Pull stocking upward to knee or groin. Make sure there are no wrinkles. Perform ending procedure actions.		

INSTRUCTOR'S SIGNATURE _____ DATE _____

COMPETENCY CHECKLIST 51:
ASSISTING WITH A STERILE PROCEDURE

ACTIONS	SATISFACTORY	UNSATISFACTORY (COMMENTS)
Perform beginning procedure actions. On clean and dry table, first open the flap that is away from you.		
Open side flaps.		
Open flap closest to you. Only touch outside of package.		
Open other sterile items and drop onto field.		
Drop them into the middle of the field.		
Once all supplies are prepared, put on sterile gloves. Open package of gloves away from field, touching only side flaps.		
Pick up one glove by the cuff and put it on.		
Place fingers of gloved hand under cuff of other glove and slip other hand into it.		
Pull glove onto your hand. Gloved hands can touch each other. Adjust gloves. You can now touch items on field. Perform ending procedure actions.		

INSTRUCTOR'S SIGNATURE _____ DATE _____

COMPETENCY CHECKLIST 52: GIVING POSTMORTEM CARE

ACTIONS	SATISFACTORY	UNSATISFACTORY (COMMENTS)
Perform beginning procedure actions. Open the morgue kit. Wear gloves.		
Position shroud under deceased with pad under buttocks.		
Apply chin strap to keep mouth closed.		
Use ties to fasten wrists and ankles together. Place gauze padding under ties.		
Fill out 3 identification tags. Place first tag on right big toe.		
Fold shroud around body. Use long ties or tape to hold it closed. Fasten second tag to outside of shroud and third tag to bag with deceased's belongings. Transport deceased to morgue. Perform ending procedure actions.		

INSTRUCTOR'S SIGNATURE _____ DATE _____

Chapter 20: Caring for the Patient at Home

VOCABULARY

agency
clutter
diaper area
discharge planner
formula

handy
imminent
indefinitely
laundromat
perishable

prewash cycle
pureed
recycling

HOME HEALTH CARE IN THE UNITED STATES

Vocabulary Sentences

1. A home health care **agency** supervises home health care workers.
2. Clients with chronic illnesses may need home health care **indefinitely**.
3. The **discharge planner** may recommend home health care for a patient.

Writing

Write a paragraph about being a home health aide. Explain why you think you would or would not like to be a home health aide.

_____

_____

_____

_____

_____

_____

_____

_____

_____

_____

_____

_____

DELIVERING HOME HEALTH CARE

Vocabulary Sentences

1. The **diaper area** on an infant should be washed at each diaper change.
2. Mrs. Jeffries doesn't like the home health aide to move any of her **clutter**.
3. People who do not have a clothes washer in their homes can do laundry in a **laundromat**.
4. The **prewash** cycle on washing machines can be used to rinse out heavily soiled items before washing.
5. Milk, meat, and other **perishables** must be kept refrigerated.
6. Infants who do not drink breast milk need to drink **formula**.

Listening

Listen to the following sentences. One word in each sentence is incorrect. Draw a line through the incorrect word and write the correct word on the line before the sentence.

_____ 1. Home health care is used to sharpen hospital stays.

_____ 2. The client is not exposed to pathogens and may be more likely to get infections.

_____ 3. Nurses, therapists, and social workers all promote home health care.

_____ 4. To be a home health aide you need to give confidence in your skills.

_____ 5. If a client is incontinent, you may give him a shampoo in bed.

_____ 6. The culture and language of the client will affect the food she chooses to eat.

_____ 7. Although a home health aide cannot give medications, he may assist the patient in breaking her own medicine.

_____ 8. Oral communication of treatments, problems, or observations must be instructed in addition to the written record.

SAFETY IN THE HOME

Vocabulary Sentences

1. All homes should have a fire extinguisher kept **handy**.
2. When death seems **imminent** the home health aide calls the home health agency.

Short Answer

Answer the following question in the space provided.

1. You are working in a client's home and you hear the smoke alarm. There is a large fire in the kitchen. There is some smoke in the rest of the apartment. List 3 things you should do. List 2 things you should not do.

Do
1. _____
2. _____
3. _____

Don't
1. _____
2. _____

Role Play

1. Choose a home health aide, a supervisor, and a client for this role play. A home health aide arrives to work in a home and discovers there are no fire alarms or a fire extinguisher. The home health aide will be shopping and cooking for the client. Role play a conversation with the client and then later with the supervisor.

2. Choose a home health aide and a supervisor for this role play. Decide on an emergency situation. The home health aide calls the supervisor on the telephone to report an emergency situation that occurred at the client's home. Describe what happened, what you did, and what help you need.

LANGUAGE AT WORK

Helena: Good morning. My name is Helena Rothberg. I'm the home health aide from the Peterson agency. This is my identification card.

Mr. Jackson: Please come in. The home health nurse told me to expect you this morning. I'm not sure how I feel about someone taking over in my house.

Helena: Mrs. Jackson, I'm not here to take over. I'm here to help you and your husband while he's recovering from his surgery. I hope that we can work together to take care of your husband. You could help by telling me some of his likes and dislikes.

Mr. Jackson: You're right, it has been a little difficult for me to do everything myself. I think he would very much like to eat breakfast in the kitchen instead of in bed. Come in and I'll show you to my husband's room.

Helena: Hello, Mr. Jackson. How are you this morning?

Mr. Jackson: Not too bad. I hope that you'll be able to help me get up out of bed. It's been hard for my wife to manage everything.

Helena: That's why I'm here. I'll help you get up to the bathroom. Then, if you like, you can get dressed and have your breakfast in the kitchen. Does that sound good to you?

Mr. Jackson: Sounds great! I haven't been into the kitchen since I got home from the hospital. I just hope I can make it.

Helena: We'll take it nice and slow. Let's start by sitting on the edge of the bed.

Questions

1. Why does Helena take out her identification card?

_____

2. What does Mrs. Jackson think the home health aide is going to do?

_____

3. Why is it important for Mr. Jackson to try to walk into the kitchen?

_____

COMPETENCY CHECKLIST 53: GIVING THE CLIENT A SHOWER

ACTIONS	SATISFACTORY	UNSATISFACTORY (COMMENTS)
Perform beginning procedure actions. Help client step over edge of tub by holding onto safety bars.		
Client may sit on shower chair. Use handheld shower to bathe client. Perform ending procedure actions.		

INSTRUCTOR'S SIGNATURE _____ DATE _____

COMPETENCY CHECKLIST 54: GIVING THE CLIENT A SHAMPOO

ACTIONS	SATISFACTORY	UNSATISFACTORY (COMMENTS)
Perform beginning procedure actions. Roll 1 towel and place around client's neck.		
Roll other 2 towels lengthwise. Place large trash bag around them and under client's head. Let trash bag hang into bucket on floor.		
Pour warm water from pitcher on client's head to wet, shampoo, and rinse hair. Protect eyes with washcloth. Perform ending procedure actions.		

INSTRUCTOR'S SIGNATURE _____ DATE _____

COMPETENCY CHECKLIST 55: GIVING AN INFANT A BATH

ACTIONS	SATISFACTORY	UNSATISFACTORY (COMMENTS)
Perform beginning procedure actions. Fill tub with a few inches of 100° to 105°F water. Talk to infant, lower her into water. Support head and neck by holding one hand under infant's arm. Wash face, then rest of body.		
Lay infant on towel and dry well. Put on clean diaper and clothes. Perform ending procedure actions.		

INSTRUCTOR'S SIGNATURE _____ DATE _____

COMPETENCY CHECKLIST 56: CLEANING IN THE CLIENT'S HOME

ACTIONS	SATISFACTORY	UNSATISFACTORY (COMMENTS)
Keep all cleaning supplies together. Take them to room to be cleaned.		
Try to reduce amount of clutter.		
Use disinfectant cleaner to wipe bathroom sinks, tubs, and toilets daily.		
Clean kitchen after each use. Floor may be cleaned weekly or as needed.		
If the client has an infectious disease wash dishes in hot soapy water and keep dishes separate.		
Dust before vacuuming.		

INSTRUCTOR'S SIGNATURE _____ DATE _____

COMPETENCY CHECKLIST 57: FEEDING AN INFANT

ACTIONS	SATISFACTORY	UNSATISFACTORY (COMMENTS)
Perform beginning procedure actions. Sit with infant comfortably. Tilt bottle so formula fills nipple.		
After 2 or 3 ounces, place infant in you lap and pat back to help her burp. Continue feeding and burping until formula is finished or until she does not want any more.		
After feeding, place infant in crib on her side. Place rolled blanket at infant's back. Perform ending procedure actions.		

INSTRUCTOR'S SIGNATURE _____ DATE _____

COMPETENCY CHECKLIST 58: SAFETY IN THE HOME

ACTIONS	SATISFACTORY	UNSATISFACTORY (COMMENTS)
Keep stairs clean of any items.		
Client should use raised toilet seat.		
Keep emergency telephone numbers near telephone.		
Encourage client to let you take away small rugs.		
Place nightlights in bedrooms and halls.		
Turn pot handles to inside on the stove.		
Keep medicines and poisonous cleaning supplies out of reach of children and confused adults.		
Wipe up spills immediately.		

COMPETENCY CHECKLIST 58: SAFETY IN THE HOME (CONTINUED)

ACTIONS	SATISFACTORY	UNSATISFACTORY (COMMENTS)
Never put electric cords under rugs.		
Use plastic glasses and pitchers instead of glass for children or confused adults.		

INSTRUCTOR'S SIGNATURE _____ DATE _____

Chapter 21: Medical Communications

VOCABULARY

bilingual
complicated
Kardex

modern
old fashioned
world view

ABBREVIATIONS

ADL   activities of daily living
assist assistance
C&B   chair and bed

inc   incontinent
pt.   patient
TCDB turn, cough, and deep breathe

ORAL COMMUNICATIONS

What Do You Say?

It can be an uncomfortable situation to be given work you cannot finish or are not sure how to do. In both situations you should talk to your supervisor about it. Write an example of what you could say in each of the cases below.

1. The nurse assigns you a task you learned to do in school, but you have not yet done it at work. You feel uncomfortable doing it alone the first time.

    _____

    _____

2. You have had a busy day at work taking care of your patients. One of your patients was incontinent in the bed 3 times and you have spent most of the afternoon changing the patient's clothes and bed. Now you think you do not have time to bathe one of your other patients before your shift is over.

    _____

    _____

Short Answer

For each of the following nurse's orders write a note to yourself in medical shorthand in the space provided.

1. Please take vital signs on Mr. Delaney in room 402 every 4 hours. Report anything unusual to me right away.

    _____

2. Ms. Poe needs to be turned every 2 hours and observed for red areas. She is in 401. Will you take care of that Robert?

    _____

3. Mr. Sinton in room 412 needs to go to radiology this morning. Would you transfer him to a wheelchair and take him down? Find out how long they need Mr. Sinton so you can pick him up.

    _____

4. Mrs. Schneider is going home today. Please make sure that she is ready to go. When her son arrives, you may transport her to the main doors in a wheelchair. He said he would be here around 11.

_____

5. I need you to do morning care for the patients in 403 and 404. Be sure to change the linens. Let me know if Ms. Hawthorne doesn't eat her breakfast. She didn't eat anything last night and I want to make sure she gets some nourishment today.

_____

Role Play

Choose a nurse and a nursing assistant for this role play. The nurse gives orders and the nursing assistant shows that he understands what he needs to do. The nursing assistant will also write a note to himself about what he should do. He may write on a paper or on the board.

NURSING ASSISTANT AS INTERPRETER

Vocabulary Sentences

1. Communications in a health care facility can be **complicated**.
2. It may be difficult for someone from a different culture and **world view** to understand what is happening in a medical facility.
3. Many health care institutions use **bilingual** staff members as interpreters.
4. **Modern** health care workers must listen to the **old-fashioned** beliefs of their patients.

Discussion Question

1. Have you ever been asked to interpret? How did it feel? Try to imagine being asked to interpret in a medical facility. How do you think you would feel?

Listening

Listen to the following sentences. In each sentence one word will be different. Draw a line through the incorrect word and write the correct word on the line before the sentence.

_____ 1. Interpreters are used in clinical settings to help take medical facilities.

_____ 2. When interpreting you should make your full attention to the patient.

_____ 3. To do a good job of interpreting you need to understand the immediately situation so you can explain it.

_____ 4. Interpreters should remind the patient that everything will be kept continental.

_____ 5. You should translate everything that is said, even if it seems unimportant to you.

_____ 6. Explain medical words carefully to the doctor so he can understand the situation.

_____ 7. Share your clinical knowledge with the doctor to help her understand the patient better.

_____ 8. Do not add anything to what is said unless you make it clear that you are starting for yourself and not translating.

WRITTEN COMMUNICATIONS

Vocabulary Sentences

1. Check the **Kardex** daily for new information on your patients.
2. The **ADL** form is a record of the care that is given to the patient each day.

Skills Practice

1. Look at the Kardex in Figure 21–1. Fill out the written assignment form below the Kardex for a nursing assistant who is working the day shift. Be sure to include everything he needs to do for the patient and at what time. Do not include information that does not concern a nursing assistant.

DIET Nourishments AM ____ PM ____ HS ___	ACTIVITY Bedrest ✓ Turn q _2h_ Up ad lib ____ TCDB ✓	Amb ____ Amb c̄ assist ____ C&B ____	PERSON TO NOTIFY Anna Callaway 236–0339	ALLERGIES Codeine
I&O ✓ Strict ____ Restrict to ____ Force ✓	BATH Total ✓ Assist ____ Self ____	RESTRAINTS Wrist ____ Posey ____ Only hs ____	TREATMENTS: D/C <u>ROM arms/legs BID</u> <u>Pressure ulcer care q8h-done RN</u> <u>Fleets PRN</u>	

VITAL SIGN TPR QID ____ BID ✓ q4 __ Oral ____ Rectal ____ BP QID ____ BID ✓ q4 __ Apical pulse ✓ Report T _≥100_ Report BP _≥180_ 100	SAFETY LOC _semi-conscious_ Seiz. Precautions ____ Siderails ↑↑ HOH ____ Vision impaired ____ Aphasic ✓ Non-Eng. Speaker ____ Geri-chair ____	____ ____ ____ ____ ____ ____ ____ ____
SPECIAL ORDERS Daily wt at ____ Blood glucose moniter at ____ Urine S&A ac ____ hs ____ q ____ Oxygen via _nc_ @ _2_ L _prn_ Mouth care q _2h_	ELIMINATION BRP ____ BRP c̄ assist INC urine ✓ feces ✓ Urinal ____ (Bedpan)/fx pan ✓ Commode ____ Colostomy ____	CODE STATUS DNR ✓ Per Dr. _Devlin_
NAME Desmond, Gladys DX CVA	DR. Devlin	ROOM 301

ASSIGNMENT SHEET				
NAME	ROOM	DX	DIET	FOOD ALLERGIES
VS				
I & O				
NOTES:				

Figure 21–1

2. Now fill in the ADL sheet for this same patient, Figure 21–2.

Name _____ Room _____

Activities of Daily Living

DATE										
I. DIET:		7-3	3-11	11-7	7-3	3-11	11-7	7-3	3-11	11-7
A. MEALS—AMT. EATEN										
B. NOURISHMENTS										
II. PERSONAL HYGIENE										
A. Complete bath										
B. Assist										
C. Self										
D. Shower/tub bath										
E. Mouth care										
F. Peri care										
G. Back care										
III. ACTIVITY										
A. Bed rest										
B. Dangle										
C. C&B										
D BRP										
E. Ambulate										
F. ROM										
IV. Elimination										
A. Bowels										
1. Amount										
2. Consistency										
3. Enema and results										
4. Incontinent										
B. Bladder										
1. Voided										
2. Catheterized										
3. Catheter care										
4. Incontinent										
V. TREATMENTS										
1. Leg exercised TCDB										
2. Anti-embol. stockings— removed and replaced										
3. Dressing changes										
4. Irrigations										
5. Soaks—hot packs, cold packs										
VI. SPECIMENS (Specify)										
VII. DIAGNOSTIC TESTS										
VIII. OTHER										
IX. SIDE RAILS UP										
X. SLEEP (naps, well, poorly)										
XI. Signature										

Figure 21–2

LANGUAGE AT WORK

A doctor receives help communicating with a patient from a nursing assistant who speaks the patient's language.

Dr. Brown: Thank you for coming to help me talk to this patient.

Juan: I'm happy to help if I can.

Dr. Brown: Good. This patient, a man, was brought into the ED last night by a stranger. He was unconscious, had a fever of 103.2, and was dehydrated. The ED staff started him on an IV and medicine to bring down the fever. Now he is awake and has pulled the IV out of his arm twice. The nurse tried to talk to him but he seems to only speak Spanish. That's why we asked you to come.

Juan: I sure hope I can help you talk to him. What do you want to talk to him about?

Dr. Brown and Juan go into the patient's room. Juan greets the patient in Spanish. (Spanish parts of the conversation are in italics. They have been translated into English so everyone can understand them.)

Juan: *Good morning. My name is Juan and I'm a nursing assistant here.*

Patient: *Oh thank God that you've come! These people are trying to kill me!*

Juan: *It must be very frightening for you to be here. But I'm here to help and so is Dr. Brown.* The patient says that he thinks you are trying to kill him.

Dr. Brown: Tell him we are trying to help him.

Juan: I did.

Dr. Brown: Good. Ask him how he is feeling.

Juan: *How do you feel?*

Patient: *I feel terrible. I am half dead. They put something in my arm that was sucking my life away. I couldn't breathe! And . . .*

Juan: *Can you wait just a minute? I want to tell the doctor what you said before I forget any of it.* He says he is half dead and that the IV was sucking his life away and making it hard for him to breathe.

Doctor: Ask him if he can breathe better now.

Juan: *Can you breathe better now?*

Patient: *Yes, of course. But there is still something in my chest, I hear it when I breathe.*

Juan: He says he can breathe better but there is something in his chest that he hears when he breathes.

Doctor: Ask him if I can listen to his chest with my stethoscope so I can hear it, too.

Juan: *May the doctor listen to your chest with his stethoscope (shows it to patient)? It is a tool to help her hear things inside your body.*

Patient: *I suppose it will be OK.*

Questions:

1. What did Dr. Brown do to show Juan that she knew he was a professional part of the health care team?

   _____

2. What did Juan do to help the patient feel more comfortable?

   _____

3. Why did Juan tell the doctor that the patient thought the IV was sucking his life away, even though he knew that an IV provides hydration?

   _____

Chapter 22: The Internship

VOCABULARY

apprenticeship
bored
corrective criticism
eager
effective

fluency
impression
initiative
intern

internship
preceptor
sense of humor

BEFORE YOU BEGIN YOUR INTERNSHIP

Vocabulary Sentences

1. The **internship** gives students a chance to practice everything they have learned.
2. An **apprenticeship** allows a nursing assistant to learn more difficult skills after the nursing assistant training is completed.
3. Right now I am an **intern** at this facility, but I hope to be a employee soon.
4. I learn so much from my **preceptor** at the internship site.

Short Answer

Look at the words "intern" and "internship." An intern is someone who does an internship. Look at the word "apprenticeship." What do you think the word is for someone who does an apprenticeship? _____

Choose the word intern or internship to complete the following sentences.

1. I am an _____ at this health care facility.

2. I am doing an _____ at this health care facility.

3. Who is the new _____ in the maternity department?

4. Kay is a terrific _____ .

5. City Hospital is a great _____ site.

What Do You Say?

Answer the following questions as you would on your first day of your internship.

1. Tell me a little about yourself.

_____

_____

2. Tell me about the program you are in.

_____

_____

3. What do you feel most confident in?

_____

_____

4. What do you think you need to learn more about?

_____

_____

_____

5. What are you going to do when you finish your internship and graduate from school?

_____

_____

_____

ON YOUR INTERNSHIP

Vocabulary Sentences

1. Journal writing is an **effective** way to improve your **fluency**.
2. Remember that people at your internship may give you **corrective criticism** to help you become a better nursing assistant.
3. Kim is a great intern, she is so **eager** to learn new things.
4. I like to see an intern who shows some **initiative** rather than just waiting for me to tell him what to do next.
5. Having a **sense of humor** makes the work day easier for everyone.
6. When I get **bored** at my internship I go to visit patients who don't have many visitors.

Writing

Begin your journal writing before your first day of your internship. Write about how you are feeling and what you are thinking about the internship. Include your hopes and expectations. Remember to write steadily without stopping to correct. Set a timer and write for 15 minutes. If you have not filled the page you may continue for another 15 minutes. Your writing should be kept in a special notebook that is used only for journal writing. Always write the date at the top of the page.

Role Play

Choose a nursing assistant intern, an internship supervisor, and a nursing assistant for this role play. The intern reports for duty on the first day of the internship. The supervisor meets the intern and explains things. The intern asks questions. The supervisor introduces the intern to another nursing assistant on the floor and they talk.

Matching

Match the internship problem on the left with the possible solution on the right.

___1. first day nerves

___2. prejudice

___3. feeling bored

___4. language difficulties

a. Tell your supervisor and your teacher.
b. Speak slowly and clearly or ask another person for help.
c. Give yourself time to get used to everything.
d. Ask for work to do. Talk to the patients. Read procedure manuals.

LANGUAGE AT WORK

This is Lucinda's first day at her internship.

Sarah: Hi. My name is Sarah. I'm a nursing assistant in this department. I don't think I've seen you before.

Lucinda: No, you haven't. My name is Lucinda. I'm a nursing assistant intern from Oak Hills Community College. I will work on this floor for the next few weeks.

Sarah: Hey, that's great. We can really use your help. Lucinda is a pretty name. What kind of a name is that?

Lucinda: Spanish.

Sarah: Really? Do you speak Spanish?

Lucinda: Yes, I do.

Sarah: That'll come in handy around here. Lots of the patients speak Spanish and it's really hard for me to talk to them sometimes. I'm trying to learn Spanish at a class here at the hospital. But it's really hard for me. Where did you learn to speak Spanish?

Lucinda: Well, I was born in Argentina and Spanish is the language of my country. I learned English in school.

Sarah: Argentina. Wow. How long have you been in the United States?

Lucinda: Almost 4 years.

Sarah: Boy, your English is really good. Did you learn that at the community college, too?

Lucinda: Some of it. I knew some before I came here from the university in Argentina. That made it easier when I got here. But I still have trouble sometimes. I don't always understand people.

Sarah: Well, if there is anything you don't understand, just ask me to repeat it. I don't mind.

Lucinda: Thanks. Where can I find Connie Brown? She's my RN supervisor. I must report to her soon.

Sarah: She should be up at the nurses' station by now. Come on. I'll show you.

Lucinda: Thank you.

Questions:

1. What is the name of the new intern? Where is she from?

_____

2. What does it mean to "come in handy"?

_____

3. Who is learning to speak Spanish? Why?

_____

4. What will Sarah do to help Lucinda?

_____

5. What do you think Lucinda could do to help Sarah?

_____

Chapter 23: The Job Search

VOCABULARY

benefit
conscientious
current
distracting

format
impress
national origin
negotiable

phlebotomist
position
volunteer

WRITING A RESUME

Vocabulary Sentences

1. I included my **volunteer** work at my son's school on my resume.
2. A job is often called a **position** by employers.
3. I will try to be **conscientious** when I am working.
4. The **format** of a resume should include all the important information and be easy to read.

Fill in the Blanks

Choose the correct word from the list below to fill in the blanks.

application
reference

certification
resume

objective

1. A _____ is a written summary of your work and educational history.

2. A _____ is someone other than family and friends who knows you and can answer questions about what kind of a person you are.

3. Nursing assistants must continue their education as they work to keep their _____ current.

4. A job _____ is a statement of what kind of job you would like to have.

5. A job _____ is a form from the employer that you must fill out when you want to work there.

Writing

Fill out the information on the form below. Use the completed form as the outline for your resume and references.

Name _____

Address _____

Phone _____

Job objective _____

EDUCATION

Name of school _____

Address _____

Program _____

Dates of attendance _____

Name of school _____

Address _____

Program _____

Dates of attendance _____

Name of school _____

Address _____

Program _____

Dates of attendance _____

EXPERIENCE

Name of employer _____

Job title _____

Job description _____

Dates of work _____

Name of employer _____

Job title _____

Job description _____

Dates of work _____

Name of employer _____

Job title _____

Job description _____

Dates of work _____

PROFESSIONAL ABILITIES

_____

_____

PERSONAL QUALITIES

_____

_____

REFERENCES

Name _____

Position _____

Address _____

Phone _____

Name _____

Position _____

Address _____

Phone _____

Name _____

Position _____

Address _____

Phone _____

GETTING AN INTERVIEW

Vocabulary Sentences

1. When you do not know how much money a nursing assistant usually is paid you may write **negotiable** on the job application.
2. Employers should not refuse to hire someone because of **national origin**.

Skill Builder

Locate 3 possible job openings for nursing assistants in your city or town. Look in the help-wanted section of the newspaper or ask people you know at health care facilities. For each opening find out the following information.

Name of health care facility _____

Address _____

Phone number _____

Position open _____

Person to contact for interview _____

Name of health care facility _____

Address _____

Phone number _____

Position open _____

Person to contact for interview _____

Name of health care facility _____

Address _____

Phone number _____

Position open _____

Person to contact for interview _____

THE INTERVIEW

Vocabulary Sentences

1. I hope that I can **impress** the job interviewer today.
2. Job **benefits** can be as important as the salary when deciding whether the job is right for you.
3. When someone taps a pencil while talking it is **distracting** to the listener.

Writing

Look at your resume and think about what kinds of questions an interviewer might have after reading it. Write down 3 questions an interviewer would be likely to ask you. These questions should be specific for you, not something that could be asked of anyone.

1. _____
2. _____
3. _____

Now write a list of 3 questions you could ask an interviewer about a job.

1. _____
2. _____
3. _____

Role Play

Choose an interviewer and an applicant for this role play. The interviewer works at a health care facility and has a nursing assistant job available. Make up a salary, benefits, and shift. The interviewer may wish to use questions from the chapter to ask the applicant.

The applicant should be ready to answer questions and have some questions to ask as well. The role play begins when the interviewer calls the applicant into the office for the interview.

ON THE JOB

Vocabulary Sentence

1. After you have a job you will continue taking classes to keep your certificate **current**.
2. My friend is a **phlebotomist** at the hospital where I work.

Listening

Listen to the following sentences. One word in each sentence is incorrect. Draw a line through the incorrect word and write the correct word on the line before the sentence.

_____ 1. Resumes and reference lists must not have any months.

_____ 2. You cannot use friends and family supervisors as references.

_____ 3. Job openings are often copied by talking to people who work in health care institutions.

_____ 4. Job applications must be filled up clearly and completely.

_____ 5. Interviews will be more successful if you prepare for her.

_____ 6. Smiling, holding hands, and dressing nicely all help to make a good impression.

_____ 7. After an interview, it is a good idea to write a thank you note to the administrator.

_____ 8. Being on time, offering to work, and asking questions are all important parts of being a good member of the health care team.

LANGUAGE AT WORK

Jane: Good morning, Sunnyside Senior Home.

Pat: Good morning. I'm interested in the nursing assistant position that was advertised in the newspaper.

Jane: You'll need to come in and fill out an application.

Pat: Can you tell me where you are located?

Jane: Sunnyside is at the corner of Oak Street and Third. Do you know where that is?

Pat: Yes I do. Is it all right if I come in today?

Jane: That will be fine. Just come to the Human Resources Department.

Pat: OK. Thank you for your help. Good-bye.

Jane: Good-bye.

Questions:

1. Why does Pat call Sunnyside Senior Home?

_____

2. What does Jane tell Pat she must do first?

_____

3. Where should Pat go when she arrives at Sunnyside Senior Home?

_____

4. Why is Pat going to Sunnyside Senior Home?

_____

5. How did Pat find out about the nursing assistant job opening?

_____

Appendix

ABBREVIATIONS

@	at
°	degrees
ac	before meals
ad lib	whenever the patient wants to
ADA	American Diabetes Association
ADL	activities of daily living
AFB	acid-fast bacilli
AIDS	acquired immunodeficiency syndrome
AKA	above-the-knee amputation
AM	morning
AMA	against medical advice
amb	ambulatory
assist	assistance
AP	apical
ATU	addictions treatment unit
AX	axillary
BID	twice a day or 2 times a day
BKA	below-the-knee amputation
BM	bowel movement
BP	blood pressure
BRP	bathroom privileges
c	with
cc	cubic centimeter
c/o	complain of
C	Celsius
C	correction
C&B	chair and bed
C&S	culture and sensitivity
CAD	coronary artery disease
CCU	cardiac care unit
CHF	congestive heart failure
cm	centimeter
CNA	certified nursing assistant
CNS	central nervous system
CO_2	carbon dioxide
COPD	chronic obstructive pulmonary disease
C section	Cesarean section
CT	computerized tomography
CVA	cerebrovascular accident
CVS	clean-voided specimen
daily	every day
DC	discontinue; stop
DC'd	discharged
D&C	dilation and curettage
DKA	diabetic ketoacidosis
DM	diabetes mellitus
DNR	do not resuscitate
Dr.	doctor
DRG	diagnostic-related group

ED	emergency department
EEG	electroencephalogram
EKG or **ECG**	electrocardiogram
EOE	Equal Opportunity Employer
ERT	estrogen replacement therapy
F	Fahrenheit
ft	feet
fx	fracture
geri chair	geriatric chair
GI	gastrointestinal
GTT	glucose tolerance test
h	hour
HBV	hepatitis B virus
HCA	home care aide
HCV	hepatitis C virus
HHA	home health aide
HIV	human immunodeficiency virus
HOH	hard of hearing
HS	at bedtime, when the patient goes to sleep
ht	height
HTN	hypertension
I&O	intake and output
ICU	intensive care unit
ID band	identification bracelet
IDDM	insulin-dependent diabetes mellitus
in	inches
inc	incontinent
irr	irregular
IV	intravenous
IVP	intravenous pyelogram
kg	kilogram
L	left
L	liter
L&D	labor and delivery
lab	laboratory
lb	pound
LLQ	left lower quadrant
LOC	level of consciousness
LP	lumbar puncture
LPN	licensed practical nurse
LTC	long-term care
LUQ	left upper quadrant
LVN	licensed vocational nurse
MAT	maternity
MD	medical doctor
med-surg	medical-surgical
MI	myocardial infarction
min	minute
mL	milliliter
MRI	magnetic resonance imaging
MS	multiple sclerosis
NA	nursing assistant
NAS	no added salt
nc	nasal cannula
NF	nursing facility
NG	nasogastric

NIDDM	non–insulin-dependent diabetes mellitus
NKA	no known allergies
NKDA	no known drug allergies
NP	nurse practitioner
NPO	nothing by mouth
O$_2$	oxygen
O&P	ova and parasites
OB-GYN	obstetrics and gynecology
OBRA	Omnibus Budget Reconciliation Act
OD	right eye
OR	operating room
ortho	orthopedics
OS	left eye
OSHA	Occupational Safety and Health Administration
OU	both eyes
oz	ounce
P	pulse
PA	physician's assistant
PACU	postanesthesia care unit
pc	after meals
PCA	patient care assistant
PCA pump	patient-controlled analgesia pump
pedi/peds	pediatrics
peri care	care of perineum
PID	pelvic inflammatory disease
PM	after noon
PNS	peripheral nervous system
po	by mouth
postop	after the operation
PPD	purified protein derivative
preop	before the operation
PRN	as necessary
PSA	prostate-specific antigen
pt.	patient
PT	physical therapist
PT	physical therapy
q2h	every 2 hours
q4h	every 4 hours
qh	every hour
QID	4 times a day
R	rectal
R	respiration
R	right
R-A-C-E	Remove-Activate-Contain-Exinguish or Evacuate
ROM	range of motion
RD	registered dietitian
rehab	rehabilitation
RLQ	right lower quadrant
RN	registered nurse
RR	recovery room
RT	respiratory therapist
RUQ	right upper quadrant
s	without
S&A	sugar and acetone
SC	subcutaneous
SNF	skilled nursing facility

SOB	shortness of breath
spec	specimen
SSE	soap suds enema
stat	immediately
STD	sexually transmitted disease
SW	social worker
sx	symptom
T	temperature
TB	tuberculosis
TCDB	turn, cough, and deep breathe
TIA	transient ischemic attack
TID	3 times a day
TPN	total parenteral nutrition
TURP	transurethral resection of the prostate
U/A	urinalysis
URI	upper respiratory infection
US	ultrasound
UTI	urinary tract infection
VA	visual acuity
VS	vital signs
wt	weight
×	times
X-ray	radiology
>	greater than
<	less than